£6.99

Psych~ ~n

PSYCHOLOGY IN ACTION

Psychology has a great deal to s~ ~ we can make our working lives more effective and re~ ~g: the way we see other people, how they see us, and our ability to communicate with others and achieve what we want from a situation. Starting from actual practice in the classroom, the police station, the surgery or the interviewing room, PSYCHOLOGY IN ACTION looks at the everyday working methods and concerns of particular groups of people and asks: where and how can psychology help?

BACKGROUND TO THE SERIES

This series is an amalgam of two proposals made independently to The British Psychological Society, one by Antony J. Chapman and Anthony Gale, the other by John Radford and Ernest Govier. The British Psychological Society's Books and Special Projects Group brought the teams together to work out the main principles of the PSYCHOLOGY IN ACTION series, in conjunction with the Society's Business and Publications Managers. This title is edited by Dr Paul T. Brown.

Titles in the series:

Counselling and Helping by Stephen Murgatroyd.

Classroom Control by David Fontana.

Police Work by Peter B. Ainsworth and Ken Pease.

NURSING IN THE COMMUNITY

Susan P. Llewelyn

and

Dennis R. Trent

Department of Psychology, University of Nottingham

Published by The British Psychological Society
and Methuen
London and New York

First published in 1987 by The British Psychological Society, St Andrews House, 48 Princess Road East, Leicester, LE1 7DR, in association with Methuen & Co. Ltd, 11 New Fetter Lane, London EC4P 4EE, and in the USA by Methuen, Inc., 29 West 35th Street, New York NY 10001.

British Library Cataloguing in Publication Data

Llewelyn, Susan
Nursing in the Community. — (Psychology in action)
1. Community health nursing — Psychological aspects
I. Title II. Trent, Dennis III. British Psychological Society IV. Series
610.73'43'019 RT98

ISBN 0–901715–57–3
ISBN 0–901715–56–5 pbk

Printed and bound in Great Britain by A. Wheaton & Co. Ltd, Exeter
Whilst every effort has been made to ensure the accuracy of the contents of this publication, the publishers and authors expressly disclaim responsibility in law for negligence or any other cause of action whatsoever.

Contents

Chapter 1   The Skills and Demands of Nursing in the Community   1

Chapter 2   Community Nursing with Elderly People   6

Chapter 3   Nursing the Handicapped   21

Chapter 4   The Special Needs of Special Patients   38

Chapter 5   Death and Bereavement   53

Chapter 6   Families in the Real World: The problems of disruption   69

Chapter 7   Sex and the Patient   83

Chapter 8   Parenting Problems   98

Chapter 9   When Things Go Wrong: The problem of child abuse   113

Chapter 10   Stress and the Nurse: A daily encounter   128

Chapter 11   When the Batteries Go Flat: The problems of burnout   145

Chapter 12   The Professional Nurse: Working together and alone   161

Index   179

Chapter 1

The Skills and Demands of Nursing in the Community

Imagine the following situations.

- You are on your own, sitting in your car, outside the house of your next patient, sorting out your case notes. Suddenly the door flies open, and the cat, looking somewhat the worse for wear, is kicked out of the door to the sound of a child screaming and an adult's voice yelling, 'And if you ever do that again, you horrible little brat, that's what's going to happen to you!'

- You are sitting by the bed of an elderly patient. You know him well, having nursed both him and his wife through a number of minor illnesses and surgical interventions. But now, your patient's problem is more serious. He turns to you, feeling for your hand. With tears rolling down his cheeks, he asks you to explain to his wife that he knows he is dying.

- You are in a staff meeting, and one of the team members suddenly gets up and rushes out of the room in a flash of temper, saying that she simply can't and won't cope any more. As she is a friend of yours, everyone in the meeting looks to you to explain what is going on. To be perfectly honest, all you really want to say is that you know exactly how she feels. But you don't think it would be 'professional' to say that, so find yourself making a number of rather lame excuses for her.

- You are in the home of a patient who has just heard the news that her much longed-for baby is severely mentally handicapped. She angrily turns to you and blames you and 'all those incompetent doctors' for what has happened, and then suddenly bursts into uncontrollable floods of tears.

These are typical of the situations that nurses working in the community face on a regular basis. But they are not the kind of situations which are normally described in textbooks. Nor are they usually mentioned in job advertisements. The skills needed to deal with them are not those that can be achieved by following straightforward nursing procedures. They are skills that can only be developed by understanding the emotions experienced by human beings, especially when they are under the pressures of illness, anxiety, fear of the future and doubt.

A competent nurse in the community has to have some way of responding to these emotions if patients are to be helped as people, not just patients. This book aims to help you to begin to make sense of these aspects of human behaviour, so that situations like the ones just described no longer seem quite so difficult to cope with. Rather than a textbook on psychology or on nursing, this is an 'ideas' book with a number of pointers to help you survive on a day-to-day basis in the business of being a nurse and managing and helping people in difficult situations.

THE SCOPE OF THIS BOOK

Nursing in the community *is* difficult, as the contents page shows. This book looks at the emotional and psychological aspects of terminal illness; mental and physical handicap; ageing; and at aspects of life which affect many of our patients, including stress, sexual relationships and parenting and its problems. In all of these chapters, our starting point is always that an understanding of how people feel is vital if you want to help them properly.

But this book is not only about other people. Nursing in the community involves a minimum of two people, both of whom are involved with each other. One is the patient, the other is you. So if you want to understand what goes on in interactions between people, you also have to spend some time on self-understanding. This does not mean you have to go in for endless self-analysis, but it does mean that you have to look at your own behaviour and feelings and see how they can affect your relationships with other people. Because of this, we have included two chapters specifically concerned with nurses themselves. Chapter 11 looks at the problem of burnout in nursing, and Chapter 12 looks at the profession of nursing. In both chapters we examine how nurses relate to each other, as well as to their patients.

A number of themes run through this book:

1. People are more than bodies

Nursing care is really only effective if the psychological aspects of people are given at least as much attention as the physical. People are obviously much more than just bodies. How they react emotionally and personally is often much more important than most of us normally think. For example, the course of recovery from an operation, or learning to cope with a handicap is very considerably affected by how a person thinks and feels. Ignoring a patient's 'personhood' means that you are giving them less than adequate care. But recognizing their 'personhood' means that you have to talk to them, and explain things to them, and listen to what they have to say. If you do not, you might as well be nursing a sick animal or a broken machine.

2. People are different

The second theme is that each patient has to be seen as an individual, and that it is wrong to assume that all people want and need the same thing. Just because *you* feel and think in a particular way, it does not mean that someone else will too. Nor does it follow that because your last patient coped in a certain way, the next one with the same condition will do the same. You really do have to assess each person afresh.

Having said that, there are obviously some things which most people have in common. So a balance has to be struck between inventing the wheel again every day and allowing someone the time and space to be different. Likewise, all nurses are individuals, and have their own unique personalities, strengths and weaknesses. You probably do not like being treated as if you are just a cog in a machine, any more than patients do. If you are to be an effective 'person manager', you deserve to spend some time thinking about yourself and your own individual values and needs, as well as understanding your patients.

3. Understanding is good for you

The third theme is that nursing in the community is demanding. It is a stressful job and requires both physical and emotional energy. But we believe that few things are as exhausting as uncertainty and ignorance, and that not knowing why people do things is a major source of anxiety and stress. Therefore, learning more about your patients and about yourself can only serve to help to reduce some of that unpredictability and stress. Ignorance is not bliss. It is an invitation to fear and uncertainty. In addition, it is an invitation to powerlessness, as you cannot really influence and control what you do not understand.

TREATING PEOPLE IN CONTEXT

Our key underlying theme is that patients are best understood and treated as 'whole people' within their social contexts, rather than as isolated bits which may need 'fixing' when things go wrong. This means two things:

- Firstly, that patients have to be seen primarily as people, and only then as having certain symptoms or problems with which they may need some expert help.

- Secondly, how people behave and feel in sickness and distress can only really be understood if you also know about their current life situations and what their background is. Different expectations, values, religious beliefs and types of family support mean that things which may only be a minor inconvenience for one person may create a very serious problem for someone else.

Spend some time trying to see what life is like from inside your patient's head, or wearing your patient's shoes. Then you may understand what your patient's difficulties and feelings actually are, and how best you can be of help. No man is an island. People cannot be understood outside the contexts in which they live.

Despite the fact that we are dealing with serious issues, we hope that you will enjoy reading from a fresh perspective; and that in being enjoyable this view will also be informative. Perhaps you will recognize situations that you know only too well, and be able to gain some new insights into the behaviour of the people with whom you work every day. Perhaps also you will gain some insight into yourself which will give you more confidence in dealing with the day-to-day challenges of nursing in the community. In the end knowledge brings understanding, and understanding brings both compassion and effectiveness.

Suggestions for further reading

French, P. (1983) *Social Skills for Nursing Practice*. London: Croom Helm.
Chapters outline some of the basic skills needed for communication with patients. Other chapters cover counselling and assessment skills.

Hall, J. (1982) *Psychology for Nurses and Health Visitors*. Leicester: The British Psychological Society/Macmillan.
This volume covers much of the same ground as our book, but provides more detail on the research findings in the area and is written in a more academic style. Recommended for anyone who finds this book interesting and wants to know more.

Tschudin, V. (1982) *Counselling Skills for Nurses*. London: Balliere Tindall.
A readable guide for community and ward-based nurses, which looks at essential counselling skills but also discusses self-knowledge and the need for support.

Chapter 2

Community Nursing with Elderly People

About one in seven of the total population is over 65. By the end of this century, the total number of elderly people is going to increase by at least a quarter. Services which are stretched at the moment are going to be even more severely stretched as the birth rate falls and the number of elderly people relying on the young grows.

Government policy over the past few decades has been directed towards providing care for the elderly in the community. As a consequence, community nurses are at present in the front line of the services provided for older people. Almost certainly, nurses in the community are going to be among the first of the professionals to face the challenges of this increased demand. In this chapter, we look at the process of ageing from a psychological point of view and consider how this could help in the care of elderly people as provided by community nurses.

THE IMPORTANCE OF INDIVIDUALS: NOT EVERYBODY WANTS TO PLAY BINGO!

First, a few words about both the process of ageing, and the services provided for the elderly. As we repeatedly point out in this book, in all aspects of community nursing it is a mistake to treat people as a group without paying attention to the individuals who make up that group. Thus it is wrong to assume that all people over the age of 65 grow older at the same rate, or that all elderly people are in need of specialist medical or nursing care. There are considerable differences between individuals: some people seem old at the age of 60, while others appear to be as young and active at the age of 85 as they were 20 or 30 years previously. Healthy and active 70-year-olds are sometimes highly amused to be approached by flag-sellers on collecting days, asking for contributions for 'old age pensioners'. But others look worn out and weary at the age of 55 or so, and are simply longing for retirement. So it is wrong to make too many assumptions about people simply on the basis of their chronological age.

It is also an error to assume that the services which do exist are equally suitable for all the elderly. The services which are provided have to be matched to each individual. For example, some older people welcome the idea of going along to a day-care centre where there is plenty of company and organized sessions of bingo or general knowledge quizzes. To others, who hate the idea of organized fun, and who have never enjoyed mixing, such an idea would be dreadful. It would not be easy and perhaps quite inappropriate to press the retired wife of a General whose idea of recreation is opera and evening classes in philosophy to go along and join in a game of cards with people with whom she has never mixed before. Equally, it would be unfair to expect an elderly man who has always been very independent and self-reliant to settle happily into a well-organized community home where he is obliged to share a room with a stranger. Yet these things are sometimes done because of a lack of attention to the person behind the label 'elderly person'. Maintaining dignity in old age is about maintaining individuality.

Community nursing for the elderly has to take into account these differences between people: it is a matter of respecting the wishes and uniqueness of each patient and not assuming that their age is more important than their personalities or preferences. This is the main message of this chapter.

UNDERSTANDING THE PROCESS OF AGEING

Becoming old is not something that happens overnight. In a sense it is true to say that we are all growing old from the moment that we are born. Throughout our lives our bodies are gradually wearing out. Our desire and capacity to learn new things is also decreasing. There is without doubt some decline in our abilities: old people are not as agile, either mentally or physically, as young people are. By around the age of 65, just under one out of every three people needs some sort of assistance with transportation or self-care. This increases to two out of every three by the age of 85. But it must also be remembered that many people remain physically active until they die. Many a grandmother can be seen energetically playing tennis or cricket with her grandchildren during school holidays. Eighty-year-olds have even been found in the ever-increasing band of marathon runners. In addition, many elderly people remain sexually active until their death and there is no reason at all why they should not do so. Indeed, the lack of sexual activity may be an early signal of depression or some physical illness.

It is true, however, that people do tend to suffer from an increasing number of minor physical illnesses as they grow older, and they may also take longer to recover from infections or injuries. Their sense organs are likely to deteriorate, so that an elderly person may well have to put up with hearing difficulties, loss of vision and loss of taste. This in turn can lead to loneliness, irritability or a number of minor psychiatric problems.

Mentally, some deterioration does take place in many people, although the degree probably depends on the individual's original level of ability. Although an elderly person may be as able to solve a problem as accurately as a young person, it will often take longer. Elderly people are often forgetful, confused and absent-minded, and of course some elderly people suffer from dementia or one of the progressive brain diseases, leading eventually to death. But all of these things are made much worse by social, psychological and economic problems, which in a way have nothing to do with the physical process of ageing. We now explore each of these in turn.

Social and psychological aspects of ageing

We live in a fast-moving, highly mobile, competitive society. This has at least two serious consequences for the elderly:

- the pace of life is much faster than it was a few years ago, let alone when the elderly of today were young

- the elderly have to learn to adapt to more and more changes, just when they are least willing or able to do so.

Next time a television programme is shown from as recently as the 1960s, have a look at the speed of movement of the camera shots: everything was much slower and simpler then than now. Speed seems to be crucial nowadays, and speed is one thing that elderly people find increasingly difficult.

In numerous ways the pace of life causes an enormous number of problems to the elderly, ranging from the serious to the apparently trivial. For a start, people talk too fast and they want decisions made quickly. The push-button traffic lights, which are designed to help people cross roads safely, do not take into account how long an elderly or disabled person takes to cross a road. Supermarkets do not allow elderly people time to pack up their purchases at the check-outs before pushing the next customer's goods down the chute. Bus conductors get impatient when it takes a while for arthritic fingers to find the bus pass in a cluttered handbag. Fashionably-dressed young shop assistants look bored when an elderly person cannot decide between two different styles of shoe, both of which are equally uncomfortable. Small wonder that elderly people sometimes feel panic at the thought of going out shopping or visiting friends. The sense of being too slow for everything can very easily lead to anxiety or depression.

Perhaps even more distressing for an elderly person is the feeling of being worthless. If you have spent a lifetime being a respected and valued employee or an important member of the local community, it can be devastating to discover that those around you suddenly seem to disregard your opinions. It is extremely hurtful suddenly to become a 'non-person' in the eyes of your society.

Mrs Owens used to be the deputy headmistress of a primary school, with a considerable amount of responsibility for its successful running. She was also an important figure in her local community, being on the management committee of a couple of local charities. When she retired, she continued to contribute to the school as a volunteer teacher, and also took on a job as co-ordinator of the school fund-raising activities. After a few years, she had a short period of illness and was obliged to hand over these responsibilities to someone else. When she regained her health she was distressed to find that she was not asked back onto the charity committees, and the school made it clear that her services were no longer required there either. It was pointed out that it was only fair to 'make way for younger people'. She was also told that she should take it easy since she had, after all, earned a rest.

This well-meaning advice upset Mrs Owens considerably, and shook her self-confidence quite a lot. Over the next few months she became painfully aware that people in the village were less and less likely to ring her up when they wanted advice on some local matter. She seemed not to be as 'important' a person as she had been. Even the shop assistants seemed to be less polite to her than they used to be. In time Mrs Owens even found it hard to believe she did have anything to contribute: she suspected that the verdict of her community was right. She was, as they implied, a useless old woman, who could not think or act as quickly as the younger people around her. She was on the verge of losing her self-esteem — the sense of self-worth that is so important for mental health.

The value and cost of experience

This sense of not being valued comes mainly from the belief that elderly people do not have anything useful to contribute to today's concerns because what they know seems to be 'out of date'. With the growing importance of computers, it may even seem that the generations no longer even speak the same language. Yet many elderly people have had extensive experience which could benefit younger people. 'New' is not necessarily better, despite what advertisements tell us. One of the main differences between an 80-year-old and an 8-year-old is that when you are 80 you have a lot of experience behind you. This experience has both advantages and disadvantages. You know a lot about the world, which gives you the advantage of having a number of skills to draw on, and the confidence that generally comes with growing up. There is a lot you could contribute, such as your memories of how things used to be done, and how people learn to work out their relationships with each other. In particular, older people can help younger people to avoid making some of the mistakes that they made. In this way, the older generation can keep younger people from having to 'invent the wheel' again.

On the other hand, the experience that older people have can also get in the way of new learning, and can make them unwilling to bother with anything new. They can start to rely too much on the past, and forget that one of the secrets of a psychologically healthy life is to keep on learning and being interested in things, right up until death. It is probably this reliance on old skills and memories which often makes young people so intolerant of the old, and vice versa.

Retirement: The time of your life?

Another problem faced by elderly people lies in the expectations which they may hold about getting old. In many ways, how we live in old age is simply a continuation of how we have lived during the rest of our lives. You do not stop being you on your 65th birthday, or on your 85th, for that matter. So the kind of things that bothered you or interested you when you were young are quite likely to be the same as those that bother you or interest you when you are old. The problem comes when you expect there to be a miraculous change when you get old. For example, many busy working people imagine that retirement will be a wonderful, extended holiday, when the sun will always shine, and they will be able to do all the things that they always wanted to do during their working lives, but never had time to do. But, instead, some working people find retirement a terrible shock as they are faced with an apparently endless future of empty days.

An additional problem can crop up when a couple who have lived together in reasonable harmony, largely because they have not actually seen very much of each other in the course of busy working lives, are suddenly forced into each other's company for 24 hours a day. Couples might not see much of each other because of shift-work patterns, or the demands of child-rearing, and this separation may in fact have been developed deliberately, as a way for the couple to stay together despite marital problems. On retirement, the couple may find they no longer have any shared interests, and actually do not like each other very much. This is probably not what they expected of retirement or old age, which then comes as a considerable shock.

Reactions to becoming older

One set of expectations that often works against elderly people getting the most out of their old age is the belief that their health or sense organs 'should' decline. Therefore symptoms or problems are sometimes ignored, although remedies are at hand.

George, a 70-year-old retired bakery worker, was having increasing difficulty in seeing, and was becoming more and more irritable at home. It was only because of persuasion from the health visitor who was attending to George's disabled wife that he agreed to have his eyes checked. Cataracts were quickly discovered, a couple of operations were performed, and George, equipped with contact lenses, could see again. In addition, George's wife reported that he had become his old, cheerful self again. George had not wanted to bother the doctor about his eyes, partly because he assumed that failing sight was just part of growing old, and partly because he thought his difficulties were not important enough to take up the doctor's valuable time.

The gradual realization for elderly people of their lessening importance, that other people are not really interested in their memories, and that they cannot keep up with things as they used to, can all lead to feelings of depression. Gradually, self-esteem diminishes, as happened to Mrs Owens. The worst thing to do at this point is anything which further reduces a person's self-esteem. Well-meaning interventions which make the person feel even less worthy or capable of being of any use to society can lead only to further depression. A suggestion of handing over control of life to someone else, by moving in with the family or into sheltered accommodation before it is really necessary, would be well-meaning but counterproductive.

Mark Twain once said that he wanted to live long enough to be as much a burden to his children as they had been to him! Surveys of the fears of old people have shown that the thing they dread most of all about getting old is not death or pain, but losing control and becoming dependent on others. Being able to look after yourself is a very important part of self-esteem. Therefore it is unwise to do anything which encourages dependence in an elderly person, as you may thereby be removing the self-esteem which results from independence. Unfortunately, many geriatric hospitals automatically tend to take over minor domestic responsibilities from their patients, and this can sometimes result in apathy and depression in the patients: quite the opposite of what had been intended.

Growing old can also lead to feelings of anger and bitterness. In a desperate need to hang on to things which held some value in the past, elderly people will sometimes become stubborn and hostile or suspicious, feeling sure that something very valuable is being stolen from them. Elderly people will often talk about their fears of being burgled or mugged, although they are the *least* likely section of the community to suffer from crime. Nevertheless, the fear that they are about to be robbed or mugged is very widespread. This fear comes not only from an awareness of how defenceless they are and how frightening such an event could be, but also from an unconscious fear, symbolically expressed, of losing something even more precious, like self-respect or life itself. In offering reassurance it helps to know that the fears, however real, may in fact be without an objective basis, yet are a means of communicating about all sorts of actual and impending losses.

Such fears and problems are of course added to by the fact that friends are likely to have died. Most importantly, a spouse may have died, leaving the survivor alone, with neither company nor practical support. Acute loneliness can result, made worse by the fact that the person may be unwilling or unable to travel to visit the friends and relatives who are still alive. The business of grieving can take many years. In consequence, many elderly people will be suffering quite acutely from the loss of loved ones at precisely that period in their lives when they have relatively few other things to do, or friends to talk to, as sources of help in their distress.

A final point which needs to be considered in understanding what is happening socially and psychologically to an elderly person is that elderly people are quite often obliged to move away from their homes, just when moving is most traumatic. The move may be into an old people's home, or it may be into the home of a relative. In either case it will involve the elderly person leaving familiar territory, and possibly abandoning possessions which may have meant a lot in the past. One local authority home known to us permits a new resident to bring only one carrier-bag-full of possessions into the home, because of restrictions of space. One sad carrier-bag is not much into which to pack a lifetime. Old age is exactly the time of life when an elderly person needs to have familiar objects around and when moving is most stressful.

Economic aspects of ageing

With the shift towards an increasingly elderly population, economic and social questions are becoming more acute. Although most working people will have contributed throughout their lives to their old age pensions and health care by means of pension and national insurance schemes, and perhaps through private saving schemes as well, it is becoming obvious that the sums thus provided are simply not enough. This is partly because of inflation; partly because of the falling number of young people now working; and partly because improvements in health care mean that more people are living into their 80s and 90s. These are the people who make the most demands on the health and social services.

So who is going to pay for the care needed by the elderly who are no longer working and earning money for themselves? In times of economic stringency or under political philosophies which stress self-reliance, all of the health and social services are threatened. While services are being reduced for all sections of the community, the elderly lack the influence to get their share (although some efforts have been made recently in this direction, as in, for example, the establishment of a 'trade union' for pensioners).

Thus provision of care for the elderly in the community, which sounded such a good idea when it was first introduced, has increasingly come to mean care by other elderly relatives, or care in private nursing homes. Sometimes carers are as old or as disabled as the elderly person who is referred to the community nurse. Some nursing homes are undoubtedly good, and provide high standards of care, but others are more interested in making money than in providing a good service for elderly patients. Large geriatric hospitals, for all their faults, at least provided a wide variety of services to the elderly patient, such as chiropody, occupational therapy and physiotherapy. As community nurses know, some patients in the community lack access to even very basic facilities or services. In addition, many carers are living under extremely stressful conditions, with pitifully little back-up.

A more personal economic issue is that many elderly people live on much smaller incomes than those in work. Of course, there are elderly people who have been able to save money during their working lives and who are no longer responsible for their dependents. These elderly people may well have enough money to enjoy their old age, and may be wealthier in their retirement than at any other time in their lives. But some elderly people live well below the poverty line and dislike the idea of borrowing money or living in debt, so actually put themselves in physical danger through inadequate heating and food. An added problem is inflation. People who have scrimped and saved throughout their lives and who are now a little confused about money values, may be unwilling to countenance spending what is actually a small sum, like two or three pounds, on food or fuel, if they can remember the days when two or three pounds was a week's wages.

THE CONTRIBUTION OF NURSES

As increasing numbers of elderly people become more and more in need of community nursing, the nurse will need a high level of skill to assess, communicate and counsel, as well as being a practical nurse. These skills are now looked at in turn.

Assessment

A patient's home conveys lots of information about their physical and mental health. In addition to assessing the physical health of a patient, it is equally important to try to understand the individual's view of the world and feelings about growing older. For example, is the person simply abandoning his or her interests in life, or is he or she adapting constructively to any loss of mobility and agility? Does the elderly person feel useful or wanted, and have some personal source of self-esteem, such as positive memories or current relationships, to guard against depression? Factors such as these will have an impact on mental as well as physical health.

An assessment of personal and family relationships is also important. Contrary to many people's ideas about present-day society, most elderly people are cared for by their own families rather than in institutions. This means that a sensitive assessment of the family is also required. As we point out in Chapter 6, very few families are actually the idylli havens of peace, love and security that the word 'family' may suggest. Community nurses are as likely to find themselves at the centre of family rivalries and longstanding conflicts as they are to find themselves in the midst of family devotion and loyalty. It is highly likely that mixed feelings will result when one member of the family suddenly requires additional care. It is all very well looking after a dependent baby when you are young and active, but when you are yourself in your 60s or 70s, and suddenly have to face incontinence in a spouse or parent, the task can be hard physically, emotionally and aesthetically. Some carers who have been quite happy as parents about changing babies' nappies may be quite revolted by the idea of helping a spouse or parent to deal with a colostomy. The revulsion can come as much from feelings of anger about having to take care of the dependent relative as from the nature of the task. Sensitive assessment of family relationships will often reveal this to be the case.

Incidentally, it is almost a cliché amongst those who work closely with families that no one version of a story is ever the whole truth. An accurate assessment of the family needs to take into account the perspectives of as many family members as possible. For example, whilst it may be that a patient's belligerence and hostility reflects an attempt to resist efforts by someone else in the family to 'take over', it is also possible that this is an indication of some personality change, due to the onset of a dementing process. Nurses working with families clearly need to have their wits about them. They also need to take care not to be 'seduced' by particular family members into taking a certain point of view. As soon as you adopt the view of one side or another you have lost the objectivity which is so important in making accurate and useful assessments.

Communication

The ability to communicate is central to our mental and physical health. Patients benefit enormously from knowing what is happening to them. But a number of factors combine to make communication more difficult for the elderly. No longer being able to hear properly what is said, for instance, means that every conversation is an effort. Relatives as well as professionals may give up trying to converse. This can then lead to a sense that other people do not *want* to talk to you (and to be fair, they may indeed find talking to you a bit of a strain if they have to shout all the time). Consequently, even fewer attempts are made to communicate, until you become almost completely cut off. Even worse, sounds may be heard as whispers, creating a suspicion that people are whispering *about* you, and do not want you to hear what they are saying. It can take a lot of concerned and aware effort to break this type of vicious cycle.

Try ways other than the spoken word. Most important is touch, which can be immensely reassuring to an elderly person who is often deprived of much physical contact with others. The nurse has to be aware, however, that there are some patients who hate to be touched by anyone, and these preferences should be respected. Writing things down may also help some patients.

Another factor which makes communication with the elderly difficult is that older people are often slower to grasp ideas, and will take more time in a conversation. This can be so annoying that the elderly person is sometimes kept in ignorance simply because no one takes the time or makes the effort to explain things. The community nurse may well have an important role in finding out what a patient knows about his or her illness, for example, and filling in some missing information.

Counselling

The third of the key psychological skills required by a nurse working in the community with the elderly, is the ability to provide counselling and support both for the patient and for the relatives who are caring for the patient. By 'counselling' we do not necessarily mean a formal session of psychotherapy, but we do mean rather more than something that happens between two people over a cup of tea or whilst engaged in standard nursing procedure like bathing or dressing. Counselling needs time to sit down together and agree to try to look at and understand emotional distress.

A key skill for the nurse to cultivate is that of being a good and patient listener, who is prepared to offer elderly people the feeling that they are, after all, human beings with rights and dignity. This can be done in part simply by giving time and attention, and in part by treating the patient as an adult, rather than as an overgrown and somewhat unintelligent child. Treating the elderly person with respect is crucial. A skilled nurse can do much to counteract the devaluing that does seem to happen to many elderly people, simply by asking for their opinion, listening to what the person says, and, as far as possible, responding constructively to what is said. Too often elderly people become 'infantilized' — treated as if they were children, and ignored or spoken to in a condescending way. For example, some nursing homes may decorate the walls of their rooms with pictures of teddy bears and cuddly toys, and insist that the residents are addressed by their first names only. This probably done in order to make the atmosphere seem warm and friendly, but the effect can be to make the elderly person feel demeaned and devalued.

By speaking to an elderly person with respect when carrying out even routine interactions, a nurse can help to challenge this view. For example, if the elderly person wishes to be addressed by their full title rather than by first name, then it is important to do so. By respecting this wish and using the full title, the nurse may be an important support for the elderly person in challenging feelings of helplessness and infantilization. Further, by respectful listening, the nurse can often encourage the elderly person to maintain involvement in adult concerns and interests. By treating the elderly person's worries and problems seriously, both self-respect and dignity can be maintained.

The other counselling role of the nurse is with the family. A lot of the community nurse's time may well be spent very productively with members of the elderly person's family, helping them to cope with the demands of caring. Numerous research studies have shown that the relatives of elderly patients, especially of those who are dementing, experience extremely high levels of stress. As a consequence, many carers suffer from a variety of minor psychiatric and physical complaints, such as headaches, irritability, sleep disturbances and so on. Effective counselling can help family carers to find the resources they need from within themselves.

There are no easy solutions to the problem, but it does appear to help if the carer can feel that someone, somewhere understands how difficult it all is, for the carer also often feels both isolated and undervalued. If you are visiting the carer of an elderly person you may be much more important than you imagine simply because you take interest in what they are doing and feeling. There may also be feelings of guilt which the nurse can do much to relieve.

Marjorie, a 60-year-old single woman, had been caring for her dementing mother for four years, and decided after much thought to take a short holiday. Marjorie had given up her job when her mother became ill, and now wanted to go away with one of her old work friends. She arranged for her married sister Sonia to look after their mother during the holiday. While she was away, Marjorie's mother developed some very unpleasant pressure sores, largely because of Sonia's inexperience. When she returned, Marjorie discovered her mother in considerable pain and, in addition, found that her mother was blaming her for all sorts of imaginary crimes. She immediately felt very guilty about having taken a holiday, and Sonia felt equally guilty for having allowed the pressure sores to develop. Consequently, Sonia resolved never to look after her mother again, and Marjorie resolved never to go on holiday again. The health visitor had to spend a considerable amount of time reassuring the two sisters that their actions were understandable and reasonable in the circumstances, and that neither of them need feel guilty. She also pointed out that many of their mother's accusations were totally unreasonable, and that such accusations were a symptom of the dementia.

Another form of guilt that the community nurse is likely to encounter is that which results when an elderly person does have to be taken into hospital for specialist care; or when relatives eventually have to give up the attempt to care because their own health is becoming severely strained. This guilt may well be expressed by projection, that is, instead of being critical of themselves, the relatives may be very critical of the hospital or of the nursing service. This is a way of expressing their own sense of guilt, although it should not be assumed that the relatives are doing it on purpose, or that they feel comfortable doing it. The best way to respond in these circumstances is not to become defensive and point out how grateful the relative *ought* to be, but rather the nurse should point out how good it is that the relative does care so much about the patient's welfare. It may take some doing, as the nurse may well feel that the criticisms are most unfair, but recognizing the process for what it is helps a good deal.

The nurse can also make a contribution to the family of the elderly or dementing patient as a provider of information. It is surprising how much will be tolerated or accepted by people if they simply know what to expect. Families are helped a great deal when they realize that some of the actions of the elderly person are the result of a disease process over which the person has no control, rather than being the result of obstinacy or wickedness. A number of support or mutual aid groups have been established in recent years which exist to provide encouragement and counsel for the relatives of elderly people. Find out if there are any such groups available locally and, if appropriate, recommend them to relatives.

AND NOW FOR THE GOOD NEWS: SOME CONCLUDING REMARKS

Getting old is not all bad news. In this chapter we have concentrated on the problems associated with ageing, because nurses are usually called in where there are problems, not where things are going well. But there are also a number of positive aspects of growing older, and it is important to remember these too.

For a start, when you grow old, you no longer have to worry about many of the preoccupations of younger people. Gone are the days of having to think about possible redundancy, pregnancy, adolescent spots, or school examinations. When asked, most elderly people actually say that they are glad that they do not have to go through all of those things again.

Second, to the elderly person, things in the outside world just do not seem to matter quite so much any more. There is evidence that people normally become more inward-looking as they grow older, so that they worry less about the opinions of others than they did. It may be that this is part of the process of getting ready to die. But there is often an opportunity to look back over life, and to put things in perspective. People may well find time to look at religious and spiritual questions, and may experience feelings of peace and tranquillity which were impossible earlier in life.

In addition, retirement does bring opportunities which, if taken up, can allow the last years of life to be full of interest and stimulation. There is no one around to clock you in and clock you out; no boss to insist on deadlines or overtime. Married couples may find that they have at last got time to spend with each other, while single or widowed people may embark on new romances. Elderly people who have paid off mortgages and hire purchase agreements may be better off than at any time during their lives, and will for the first time be able to take exciting long holidays in far away places. Others may take advantage of the lack of time commitments to develop new interests; for example by joining one of the evening classes for elderly people now run by numerous local authorities.

Old age, then, can be a time for both consolidation and growth. The fact that it is so often a time of difficulty and decline is in part due to our attitudes towards the elderly. Community nurses, as respected members of society, have an important role to play in encouraging a more sensitive and respectful attitude towards the elderly. To treat the elderly as useless or as unworthy of concern is not only a tremendous waste of human resources; it is also a mean and cruel measure of what our society thinks of as important. In addition, and from a more 'selfish' point of view, it is in our own interests to develop positive attitudes towards the elderly. The way we treat elderly people today will shape the way that we ourselves are treated when we, in turn, become old.

Suggestions for further reading

Brearly, C.P. (1975) *Social Work, Ageing and Society.* London: Routledge and Kegan Paul.
  Although written for social workers, this book could also be of considerable interest to community nurses. It is a readable account of the way society responds to the elderly, as well as an examination of the process of ageing.

Gilleard, C.J. (1984) *Living with Dementia: Community care for the elderly mentally ill.* London: Croom Helm.
  A clearly-written account of some of the stresses and problems likely to be experienced by families caring for elderly dementing relatives. It also provides a simple problem check-list and family strain scale which could be very useful for community nurses working with carers.

Powell, L.S. and Courtice, K. (1983) *Alzheimer's Disease: A guide for families.* Reading, Ma.: Addison-Wesley.
  Although primarily an American text, this volume will also be of general interest. It is a guide for families, clearly and sympathetically written, and has plenty of practical advice.

Chapter 3

Nursing the Handicapped

In this chapter we look at the contribution that community nurses can make to helping people who, although not 'ill' in the strictest sense of the word, do have some problem or difficulty with normal day-to-day living which is connected with some malfunction of their body or brain – the people called handicapped. In some cases, handicapped people may be referred directly to the nurse; in others a handicapped person may be living in the family of patient. In either case some understanding of the psychology of handicap may be useful in knowing how best to help the family or the individual.

The biggest difficulty in talking about handicapped people is in trying to define what a handicap is. What might be limiting to one individual may not be to another; loss of one eye may not limit a telephonist very much, but it would be devastating to an artist. Likewise, what may be restricting in one individual may not be in another; not being able to walk does not hamper your ability to enjoy music. So what does the term handicap mean? Well, we can say as a generalization that a handicap is any condition which limits or restricts a person's behaviour or potential. This means that most people, at some point in their lives, are likely to be handicapped in one way or another. However, nurses usually find themselves facing three main types of handicap during their working lives: mental handicap, physical handicap and sensory handicap. We deal with each of these areas in turn, and show how many of the problems of the handicapped actually stem from having to live with the rest of us who are not handicapped in the same way.

MENTAL HANDICAP: WHAT IS IT?

Records exist of mentally handicapped people since before 3000 BC.

21

Since that time there have been numerous different ways of coping with the mentally handicapped, some of which have been extremely cruel and some of which have been both humane and productive. Nowadays, the treatment received by the handicapped can vary between these two extremes, although downright cruelty is probably quite rare. Nevertheless, most mentally handicapped people do not receive the level of care from the education, housing or health services that most of us who are of normal intelligence can expect to receive. The mentally handicapped person is particularly reliant on the help and concern of others who are not handicapped. In some cases the mentally handicapped person is also very vulnerable to exploitation or neglect, and relies on the 'normal' people around to notice and put a stop to any such abuse.

Many people are still confused by the distinction between the mentally ill and the mentally handicapped. Broadly speaking, a mentally ill person has normal intelligence, but has experienced some difficulty in living which has led them to behave or feel in ways which are distressing to themselves or to others. In some cases they may be suffering from an 'illness' such as schizophrenia, or they may just feel very depressed or anxious. They will quite often recover and continue to live an entirely normal life. On the other hand, the mentally handicapped person will never recover from the handicap, since mental handicap is neither an illness nor a result of some difficulty in personal relationships or adjustment. The problem is one of low intelligence, giving rise to poor social skills or adjustment.

Whether someone is classified as mentally handicapped technically depends on the score they obtain on a standardized IQ test. These tests, which are normally administered by qualified psychologists, examine the whole range of abilities that might be expected of someone at each stage of life. The psychologist, therefore, looks at the kind of things that the person can do, and compares them with what others of the same age can do. If the discrepancy is too great, some degree of handicap will be suspected. For example, a child who is found to be unable to tie his own shoe laces at the age of 10 might well be classified as mentally handicapped if other evidence also supports this view, whereas a child of two clearly would not be seen in this way. Obviously, a wide range of tests has to be used, as some children will have difficulty with specific areas (like reading), which does not mean that they are handicapped in other ways. No attempt should be made to make a diagnosis on the basis of only a few tests.

But in terms of everyday living, much more important than scores on IQ tests is whether mentally handicapped people have the ability to get along in society. Do they have the social skills which enable them to make friends with other people and look after themselves? Do they have some degree of emotional stability, which means that they can live reasonably happily in a family setting? In fact, how friendly and competent are they in social situations? This is far more important in deciding their future than whether they have a particular score on an IQ test. If as a nurse you want to understand the plight of a mentally handicapped person, or of a family who has a handicapped child, then the person's IQ or diagnosis is only background information to establishing how well the person fits into the family, and how well the family fits into the neighbourhood.

Mental handicap makes people particularly vulnerable to the trials and tribulations of everyday life. It limits the ability to think things through or to use resources like information centres, libraries or further education. If intelligence is the attribute which lets human beings deal with the complexities of the world and plan into the future, then limitations of intelligence obviously limit that capability, right down to, say, the skills of maintaining personal cleanliness.

The present policy of closing down many of the large hospitals for the mentally handicapped (and for the mentally ill) means that in the near future more and more handicapped people are going to be living in the community, either with their families or in group homes. Therefore, it is becoming even more crucial that we learn how to ensure that the mentally handicapped learn to live in society, and that society learns how to live with the mentally handicapped.

What causes mental handicap?

We know what causes approximately 50 per cent of cases, but the causes of the remaining 50 per cent are largely unknown. There are five main types of cause:

1. Maternal ill-health during pregnancy.
This includes mothers who have contracted rubella during pregnancy; who have suffered from poor nutrition; or who have smoked heavily or taken a variety of drugs.

2. Environmental causes.
Children are much more than their genetic make-up at birth. If a child's early environment is impoverished, so that the child is rarely talked to or played with, then what intelligence he or she is born with will probably not be developed to its full potential. Unfortunately, it has been demonstrated that cases of mild mental handicap are much more common in

the lower social classes, suggesting that when there is a stimulating and varied environment for the child (as might be found in the homes of children with a more materially wealthy background) then the child is much less likely to grow up handicapped than when the environment is poorer.

3. Chromosomal or metabolic deficiences.
These include Down's syndrome and disorders such as PKU (phenylketonuria), some of which can be treated and some of which cannot. Some Down's syndrome children may be severely mentally handicapped, while others will be as intelligent as many normal children.

4. Trauma.
This includes brain damage at birth (as, for example, when the new-born baby has a stroke or where there is forceps damage), and brain injury caused after birth, for example by blows to the head or vaccine damage. Brain damage leading to mental handicap may occur later in life as a result of accident or injury.

5. Infection.
Some infections during life, such as meningitis and encephalitis, may also cause brain damage. The extent of the handicap will depend on the severity of the infection, the stage of development reached before the illness, and the speed with which treatment is started.

The community nurse may well encounter individuals who are mentally handicapped for any of the above reasons, or for no known cause. In any situation the first response of the nurse has to be the same: acceptance and respect of the person, in spite of any feeling of reluctance or anxiety, even though the handicapped person seems frightening or in some cases grotesque.

What can be done to help the mentally handicapped?

Recent treatment approaches for the mentally handicapped have stressed the importance of the fullest possible integration into the community, and of encouraging independence. Among other things, this means respecting the uniqueness of all mentally handicapped people, and trying to encourage them to develop their own individuality. The extent to which this is possible depends on the degree of handicap, but the goal is that every person should have a chance to develop in their own way as fully as possible. This actually means that those who take care of the mentally handicapped now have to do things a bit differently from how they did things in the past. The mentally handicapped used to be kept together in large units or wards, and much of their day-to-day care was provided for them by nurses or supervisors. The problem with this was that the mentally handicapped person tended to become dependent on the staff of the hospital or unit, so that individuality and self-reliance became almost impossible. In addition, mentally handicapped people tended to get labelled by their problems, so that any attempt to develop new skills was doomed to failure from the start. Imagine how you would feel if every time you went into town shopping you had to go in a bus which had *St Swithin's Home for the Mentally Handicapped* written all over it. You would probably feel that everyone was staring at you, knowing all about your inferiority. Not a good way to try and become integrated into the community. Yet the balance between openness and over-protectiveness is not an easy one to find.

Nowadays, many mentally handicapped people live either in their own homes with their families or in group homes with other mentally handicapped people, rather than in big institutions. There are probably dangers in this approach too, as for some mentally handicapped people the support of an institution is actually very necessary. Some families, for a variety of reasons, are unable to care for the handicapped person in their midst, so that the best solution for all concerned is for the person to be cared for in an institution for much of their life. As we have said elsewhere in this book, there is no single correct solution: each set of circumstances has to be dealt with on its own merits, though lack of resources makes this appear as a counsel of perfection at times.

But what can I as a nurse do?

Starting at the very beginning, the nurse has a particular role to play in helping prevent cases of mental handicap from ever occurring in the first place. Proper care of maternal health both before and during pregnancy would undoubtedly prevent some cases of mental handicap, and the administration of the rubella vaccine to almost all girls of child-bearing age has been a major preventive success. Being careful about drinking, smoking and drug intake is also important, and can be clearly recommended by nurses to expectant mothers.

Tragically, some parents cause traumatic brain damage in a previously normal child. This can happen if the parent physically damages the child by violent hitting or shaking. In one hospital for the mentally handicapped which we know the nurses all say that few things are more distressing than the sight of Sandy, a beautiful little girl, originally of normal intelligence, who has been handicapped for life by physical abuse at the hands of her father. She sits and smiles at everyone, but recognizes no one. It may be that at some point in your career you come across a case of suspected child abuse which you could help prevent. We discuss this further in Chapter 9.

Other cases of mental handicap can occur as a result of infections such as encephalitis or meningitis. Although some of these tragic cases are probably unavoidable, there are times when speedy medical intervention (for example, when a child suddenly develops a very high temperature) can prevent irreversible brain damage. A nurse working with children should be familiar with some of the early warning signs, such as fever and convulsions.

When mental handicap is present there are a lot of things that a nurse can do to help. Initially, it may be necessary to spend time with the parents of a mentally handicapped child to help them understand the limitations and potentials of the handicap. It is still the case that some parents are given the news about the handicap in a very casual and hurtful way. Recently a case has been reported of parents being told in a hospital corridor that their new baby was mentally handicapped by a doctor who would not stay to explain, saying he had to go off to lunch! Giving the news that a much longed-for baby is handicapped has been described as rather like carrying out an operation without an anaesthetic. Parents will need a lot of support in order to be able to grieve for the 'loss' of the normal child that they never had, and to accept and love their mentally handicapped child.

Tessa and her husband Mark had been married for about three years before they decided to have a baby. It took some time for the desired pregnancy to come about, but when it did, they were both thrilled and excited. However, when the expected date for the birth came and went, Tessa started to get worried, and although she did want to have as natural a birth as possible, agreed that the birth should be induced about two weeks later. She experienced a reasonably comfortable labour, but she very soon became aware that all was not well in the delivery room. Mark was ushered away, and the baby whisked off to the special care unit. The obstetrician eventually told Mark that the baby had suffered anoxia at birth, and that they were very lucky that the baby had not died. However, he would very probably be mentally handicapped for life.

Nobody clearly explained to either of them was happening, and Tessa was told she could go home a few days later, leaving the baby in hospital. When she and the baby were reunited in a few weeks, Tessa had immense difficulty in accepting him. Eventually she was able to confess to the visiting nurse that she was convinced that her 'real' baby had died in hospital, and that a little handicapped imposter had been substituted for her own baby. She also said that she wished the baby had indeed died. Having been able to express her feelings, without being condemned for them by the nurse, Tessa slowly began to accept what had happened, not as a punishment or as a malicious trick played on her by someone else, but simply as a tragedy. She then very slowly developed some feelings of love for her baby, and gradually come to value the child as much as the two healthy children that she and Mark had later.

It is true, fortunately, that many parents do accept their mentally handicapped children, and in the end say that their handicapped child brings them a great deal of joy. But in the short term the marital relationship may be placed under real strain as the parents seek to understand and explain to each other and to themselves what has happened to them, and learn how to cope. For single parents, or where the pregnancy was unplanned, there may be additional difficulties, as the handicap may be experienced as a 'punishment'. A nurse will have to find the time and skill in such difficult circumstances to help the parents to express and come to terms with their feelings of grief, anger and guilt, which are normal and to be expected. Ask the parents to talk about their feelings, making sure that you do not react either negatively or too positively to what they say. Instead, just show them that you are willing to listen, and will not be shocked by what they say. Give them the time to talk about their own reactions, which they may well need to do time and time again. Reassure them that certain emotional reactions frequently occur. For example, it is quite common for husband and wife to lose interest in sex for a while after the birth of a handicapped child. It will help them to know that this is not unusual. On the other hand, the nurse must also be aware that some parents will not want to talk, and respect that decision.

Sadly, some parents will find it impossible to accept their child, and seek to have the child adopted or taken into the care of an institution. For some families, and for some mentally handicapped children, this is the best solution in the circumstances.

Robert, a 17-year-old boy with Down's syndrome, had been cared for by his parents since his birth, and had in many ways been a happy and responsive child. However, as he grew older, he became more and more aware of his limitations, and how different he was from other boys, and started to express his frustrations by hitting out at his parents, and by self-mutilation. It was getting difficult to take him out anywhere, and on several occasions, Robert's mother had to go to the local casualty department because of wounds inflicted by Robert. At the same time, Robert's father suffered a series of minor angina attacks, and was warned by the family doctor to take life easier.

Robert's parents were both feeling increasingly worn out by Robert's behaviour, and with great reluctance eventually concluded that they could no longer continue to look after Robert at home, and asked for placement for him in a local authority hostel. However, their request was refused, and it was only with the help of their doctor and the community nursing service that a place was eventually found for Robert in a hostel run by a voluntary society. As soon as Robert had settled down, his relationship with his parents improved dramatically, and he was able to spend holidays with them without any problem. As Robert became more involved in the life of the hostel, his self-mutilating behaviour also diminished.

Even with the most loving of parents, there are going to be continuing life problems for the mentally handicapped individual. Many handicapped children will have difficulties with the day-to-day routines that most children take for granted, such as toileting, dressing or feeding, and being able to run simple errands. This is not the place to go into detail about some of the techniques that have been devised to help encourage the development of mentally handicapped people, except to say that specialist help is available for many of the difficulties that parents encounter. The best course of action if a handicapped person is repeatedly soiling or wetting or making no progress in self-care skills, is to arrange for resources to be brought in from the appropriate local service. Likewise, help is available to deal with the more distressing behaviour sometimes shown by mentally handicapped people, such as self-mutilation or public masturbation.

Personal and social needs of the mentally handicapped

More difficult to deal with, of course, are the social problems of being mentally handicapped. It is still the case that a lot of prejudice exists towards the handicapped, so that it is even harder for mentally hand-icapped young people to get jobs than it is for normal youngsters. Their access to housing and educational facilities is also very limited. Perhaps even more cruel than this is the attitude that some non-handicapped people have towards the handicapped, so that it is not unusual for mothers to be told that they should not bring 'that' into the supermarket or church hall. As handicapped children grow older, they are often very actively discouraged from taking part in the activities which are open to most young people, such as going to discos or youth clubs.

This brings us to another important subject, which is the wish expressed by many mentally handicapped people to be able to enjoy and express their sexuality with others, as 'normal' people can. In general, the production of children may well be very inadvisable but, with appropriate contraception, there is no good reason why many mentally handicapped people should not be able to have sexual relationships like the rest of us, if they so choose. The nurse may be an especially important person here, in helping concerned parents to come to terms with the independent development of their son's or daughter's relationships. When parents have become extremely protective towards their handicapped child they will see the sexual potential of their child as very threatening. The nurse has to help the parents to see that at some point it is necessary to let go, and allow the young person to grow up with as much independence as he or she is able to manage.

Encouraging independence does not stop with adolescence, As the person grows older, it becomes even more important to try and develop and maintain self-care skills. This is so for a variety of reasons. For a start, as the handicapped person grows up, he or she will obviously get bigger and stronger, and hence will be less easy to lift or control. Early training in toileting, self-care, feeding and communication skills will pay off in later years. But in addition to self-care skills, a strong sense of self-reliance will eventually help the handicapped person to deal with the problems which may well arise following the death or disability of parents. Bereavement is a terrible blow for most people, but it is especially distressing when you lose not only your parents, but also your home, most of your possessions and your way of life. Sadly, this is what happens to many mentally handicapped adults when their parents, who may have devoted most of their lives to caring for their handicapped child, eventually die or become disabled themselves, and there is no one left to do the caring. In such cases there is often no option but institutionalization, which is obviously most distressing for all those concerned. Knowing this, a nurse can be influential in preventing much future unhappiness by encouraging parents to talk and plan for the future when they will no longer be around to care for their children.

Mental handicap is in some ways the most devastating of all the handicaps which may be encountered during the community nurse's working life. Yet the mentally handicapped person may well not be as unhappy as other handicapped (or able-bodied) people the nurse will meet. We now to turn to consider the two main other types of handicap: the physically handicapped and the sensorily handicapped.

THE PHYSICALLY HANDICAPPED

There are numerous causes of physical handicap:

- genetically transmitted conditions
- birth trauma
- accidents and injuries
- illnesses such as polio or strokes
- complications from a variety of other disease processes.

Some of the difficulties faced by people who are suffering losses and physical limitation are considered elsewhere in this book (in Chapters 4 and 5 especially). We concentrate in this chapter on the emotions and frustrations likely to be experienced by the physically handicapped in their daily lives.

Stigma

Despite the wide variety in causes, what all the physically handicapped have in common is the fact that they have to live in a world which is dominated by the able-bodied. In consequence they are often looked down on by others because they are not 'normal'. An American sociologist called Erving Goffman has described the process by which people who are different are labelled as 'deviant', and are seen as either to be pitied or condemned, with the result that they are *stigmatized*. People can be said to be stigmatized when they try to hide or deny the fact that they have a particular illness or condition, or when others avoid or blame them for having the condition. Basically, stigma is a kind of disgrace, which gets linked by both sufferers and normal people to conditions like physical and mental illnesses or handicap.

The result of being stigmatized is that individuals feel a sense of shame for being who and what they are, as well as experiencing isolation and loneliness. A number of conditions, such as epilepsy and severe and obvious physical disabilities, are particularly prone to stigmatization. The more disfiguring or 'shameful' the disablement, the greater the stigma. For example, if because of a birth trauma or genetic defect a child has the use of only one arm, or has a prominent birthmark, that child is highly likely to be stigmatized at school, so that he or she not only has the actual problems of being physically handicapped to deal with but also the teasing and taunting of other children.

Adults may not so often be subject to teasing and taunting but they are likely to be on the receiving end of a different sort of unkindness: the sort of thoughtless unkindness which is summed up in the title of the BBC radio programme for the handicapped *Does he take sugar?* In other words, physically handicapped people are often assumed to be unintelligent and unable to think or speak for themselves, simply because of the general negative stigma attached to their physical disability. Handicapped people describe their shame and anger when the able-bodied simply fail to 'see' them in shops and other public places, or, when they do see them, either stare or look away quickly. This sort of experience inevitably makes the handicapped person's life even more difficult to bear.

Almost all handicapped people feel stigmatized at one time or another and have to find ways of coping with it. Some readily find the inner resources they need, but most disabled people will have distressing experiences at the hands of the thoughtless. The community nurse can be of great help here. Understanding the processes of stigmatization may be a first step for the handicapped person in overcoming the sense of shame. Being able to express some of the anger that handicapped people feel can be a second. A third, and very crucial step, is self-acceptance, which can only take place if the handicapped person has enough positive experiences to counter the negative ones which the world at large is likely to offer. Whilst parents or spouses are the most important people in the life of the handicapped person, and are going to be the ones who can help most, nevertheless the nurse's influence as a key professional and objective person is vitally important too.

The nurse's role

At the most basic level it is absolutely essential to relate to the handicapped individual as a person first, and the handicap second. Next, it is vital to remember that just because the handicapped person may not be able to walk or speak clearly, or may have to wear some special apparatus such as a helmet or callipers, this does not mean that he or she is unable to feel and think just like anyone else. Furthermore, it is essential to recall that 'the handicapped' must not be lumped together as a group, any more than 'the English' or 'students' can be: *each individual is an individual* and has his or her own unique needs and emotions.

Consequently each person has to be treated as an individual, not as more or less 'typical' of a group or class. The skilled nurse is one who conveys to every handicapped person a sense of value, and a sense of being accepted for what he or she is.

Social and financial problems

A number of other problems are of course encountered by the handicapped which have little to do with stigma, but are either the direct or indirect result of their physical disability. A direct consequence of some physical disabilities is restriction on mobility. Not being able to move around easily under your own steam places a considerable strain on your sense of independence and personal competence, as well as on the patience and tolerance of friends and relatives. Even if you can get hold of efficient and comfortable mobility aids such as specially adapted cars or wheelchairs, it still means that you are tied to that piece of machinery, and that every trip involves a certain amount of planning and forethought. The ability to nip out to the shops or to go for a walk on a beautiful summer's day, which most of us take for granted, is frequently only achieved after considerable effort and negotiating a number of obstacles, ranging from uncooperative staircases and sharp corners to unhelpful bus conductors and uncomfortable artificial limbs.

Added to all of this is one of the indirect consequences of handicap – most physically handicapped people are financially worse off than their able-bodied brothers and sisters. Although various allowances (such as disability pensions, mobility allowances and so on) are available to the handicapped, nevertheless many handicapped people are actually living on or below the poverty line and have very little opportunity or few resources with which to alter their circumstances. There are, of course, exceptions, and it is always possible to hear of people, such as Douglas Bader the pilot, Christy Brown the poet, President Roosevelt of the USA, or Elizabeth Browning the writer, who all overcame enormous obstacles to live astonishingly productive lives. But these are the exceptions, and it remains true that one of the major problems faced by the handicapped is in fact poverty and the tremendous social and personal obstacles that exist to doing anything very much about it.

SENSORY HANDICAPS

The third and final area is that of sensory loss. Such handicaps include blindness and deafness and, as with mental handicap, may occur either for genetic reasons or as the result of an accident or other specific event. Those with sensory handicaps face some problems unlike those in the other two groups and therefore need to be viewed separately.

The sound of silence . . .

Deafness is not at all uncommon. Approximately one in five of the population suffers from some degree of deafness, and about half of these are quite seriously afflicted. Although many people who are hard of hearing do have hearing aids prescribed for them, they are not always comfortable or effective, so people quite often do not wear them. Being deaf cuts you off from other people, and creates feelings of isolation and bad temper. As with other handicaps it also means that many of the things which most take for granted are made much more difficult.

Living with deafness

The birth of a deaf child (as is the case for all other handicaps) can be a considerable upset to the family, who have to learn a whole new set of skills to communicate with their new baby. Considerable controversy exists within the community of deaf people and their helpers about whether deaf children should be taught to lip read and, as far as possible, speak like other children, or whether they should be taught sign language first instead. There are advantages and disadvantages to both procedures. What is crucial is that the child is welcomed into the family as warmly as any other child, and that some form of communication channel is established with parents and siblings. Deafness does not mean that the person is unable to communicate; it simply means that one particular channel of communication is unavailable. With ingenuity, imagination and encouragement, families can learn to communicate with their handicapped child. Touch is an especially important medium, and games can be adapted so that touch and sight can replace auditory communication.

For those who become deaf the change and loss can take a lot of getting used to. The pleasures of music or the radio are no longer available and conversation with friends or family is increasingly difficult. No wonder, then, that some of those who go deaf also get depressed as they mourn the loss of their hearing and of many of their social contacts.

But the problem can also affect those who live or work with the deaf person. The difficulty for those who interact with the deaf is that, probably because of the stigma attached to any form of handicap, many people who are hard of hearing are somewhat ashamed of the fact, and may try to conceal their handicap. Hence they may avoid wearing their hearing aids, or even refuse to go for hearing tests. Other people then have to raise their voices in order to be heard. When conversations are routinely carried on at a high volume there is an unfortunate consequence. Normally we only shout when we are feeling angry or frightened. People who routinely have to shout at each other in order to be heard often report feeling angry or irritated most of the time, even though there is no very good reason to be angry. Hence, the general quality of relationships tends to decline. This may affect the community nurse too. If you do have to spend much time with deaf people you may sometimes find yourself feeling irritated with them. It is important to understand why, and not to blame the person, but instead to seek to find out why a hearing aid is not being worn. It may be because the aid is ineffective, uncomfortable or whistles when near other loudspeakers; or it could be because the whole idea seems shameful and stigmatizing; or in the elderly, arthritic joints may be making adjustments difficult. You will only be able to give the correct advice if you have considered all of these possibilities.

Living in darkness . . .

Being blind is perhaps one of the most disrupting handicaps, since so much of the occupational, social and entertainment world is geared towards the sighted. Books, television, easy access to public places, photographs of your family, private transport and a host of other aspects of life are less accessible or completely inaccessible to the blind. Small wonder then that many blind people feel isolated and somewhat resentful towards a world which seems to pass them by.

There is a clear link between blindness and old age. Eighty per cent of blind people are over the age of 65, so the difficulties of blindness are added to the problems of ageing. Furthermore, total blindness is comparatively rare, and most people who are labelled 'blind' do actually have some residual vision. Frequently they can at least distinguish between light and darkness. Being born blind is a fairly rare occurrence. Technically, the classification of people as blind depends on whether they can read very large print, or whether their mobility is seriously handicapped. The more problems they have in these two areas, the more likely it is that they will be classified as blind.

From an emotional point of view, having some residual vision does not seem to help the blind person. In fact, it appears that the partially sighted have more rather than fewer problems than the completely blind. This may be because partially sighted people are still trying to make the most of their limited abilities, comparing themselves with 'normally' sighted people, and feeling frustrated with failure. Experiencing gradual loss of vision (as can happen with cataracts) can be very depressing, as well as anxiety-provoking. (See, for example, the case of George the bakery worker described in Chapter 2.) Possibly, completely blind people have less upset because they do not have to keep being reminded of what is missing and also because they develop alternative sensory modalities, like hearing, more extensively in order to compensate for the loss of sight.

Keeping the blind on the move

For many blind people, being able to become or to remain mobile is crucial. Mobility is very clearly linked with independence. Being independent is linked with self-confidence and a positive self-image (see Chapter 4 for a discussion of self-image). A number of aids are available to help blind people get around, including guide dogs, special braille maps and the long cane (a more sophisticated version of the white stick). No doubt the patients whom you encounter will have been recommended one or other of these aids. But whatever aid is prescribed by the blind mobility officer (who is usually available to help), how the individual feels about his or her blindness and circumstances is the key factor in becoming or staying mobile. This is actually far more important than the 'objective' degree of handicap suffered by the patient. If a patient sinks into despair, and if relatives fail to encourage the patient to stay as independent as possible, then it is highly likely that the person will fail to learn to become mobile. However, if the family of the blind person encourages the patient to take risks, to experiment and to persist in spite of failures, then that person is far more likely to be successful in staying mobile. It may be, therefore, that a community nurse can help blind people simply by encouraging them and their families to persist with the trials and tribulations of being mobile in a world full of odd corners, rapid traffic and inconveniently placed furniture. Point out to the families that they may do more harm than good by trying to be too protective to the blind person.

Keeping the blind in touch

The other main problem faced by blind people is of course difficulty in reading. A lot of our day-to-day activities, from following recipes and finding out what is on the radio tonight, to filling in benefit claim forms and income tax returns, depend on our ability to see. Only a very small percentage of blind people can read braille, so most are dependent on the goodwill of friends and neighbours to keep them in touch with what is going on, and to help them to cope with 'officialdom'. In the health care field, this can present some special problems. For example, without special help, the blind person will not be able to read the instructions on the medicine bottle, nor be able to know which tablets to take when. If you cannot see, then the fact that the tablets are different colours will not be of much use to you. The nurse working with a blind patient has to be extremely resourceful in working out ways of dealing with problems like these, such as keeping different types of tablets in differently shaped bottles, or putting the different containers in different parts of the room. The chances are, of course, that many of your visually handicapped patients may have worked out coping strategies of their own to deal with this sort of problem, which should of course be used and built upon, and not rejected in favour of your own strategies. Some very useful tips can be obtained by looking through the newspapers published by the Royal National Institute for the Blind (RNIB).

Like the deaf individual, the blind person still has other senses which can be used for communication. Smell, touch and hearing can become very well developed in blind people and bring a lot of unexpected pleasure into their lives. But this is not to deny that the blind person may well feel an acute sense of loss, especially if the blindness has recently developed. Do not attempt to 'jolly' people out of their grief if they appear to be distressed. Rather, try and listen to their sadness. Help them devise ways of living life to the full as far as is now possible.

CONCLUDING REMARKS

Having a mental or physical handicap is bad enough. But the rest of us do not make it any easier by our response to the handicapped. We may not be able to do very much about how other people behave, but we can do something about our own behaviour. If you have never had any personal contact with a handicap or suffered any kind of handicap yourself, it is sometimes difficult to realize the pain that can be caused by stigma and rejection. Make sure you pay attention first to the person behind the handicap. By this means you will help the individual to keep a sense of worth and value, vital if all a person's remaining resources are to be mobilized in adapting to and compensating for the handicap.

Suggestions for further reading

Calnan, J. (1983) *Talking with Patients*. London: William Heinemann.
A guide to good practice when communicating with patients, with chapters on the special needs of handicapped patients, and the deaf and blind.

Newson, E. and Hipgrave, T. (1982) *Getting Through to your Handicapped Child*. Cambridge: Cambridge University Press.
Aimed at parents, this book may also be interesting to nurses who work with handicapped children. It is full of practical advice, and offers insight about both children and their parents.

Goffman, E. (1968) *Stigma: Notes on the management of spoiled identity*. Harmondsworth: Penguin.
This is the classic book on stigma and how it affects the handicapped.

Landsdown, R. (1980) *More Than Sympathy*. London: Tavistock Publications.
Aimed primarily at those concerned with handicapped children, this book is also useful in pointing out problems experienced by adults.

Chapter 4

The Special Needs of Special Patients

Throughout the course of their career, most nurses are likely to come into contact with a group of people who are somewhat special. If seen walking down the street, these people would probably not be thought of as different or special: yet they are unusual, in that they have had experiences which have made them *feel* different. Many have ongoing needs that other people do not have. Others may have had operations that have left them with changes in the way they look or carry out daily routines. For these people the *feeling* of being different is often more difficult to deal with than the *fact* of being different.

Three situations will help us to consider the kinds of difficulties that a nurse might encounter:

- the circumstances of someone who is tied to a service such as dialysis
- the problems that can arise when someone must change their daily routines, as in the case of those who have had colostomies or ileostomies
- the difficulties of those who have undergone body changes, as in the case of a mastectomy.

Besides *feeling* different, these people are special because in many cases the nurse may be one of the very few people outside the family to be aware of the situation. Because of this the nurse is especially important in helping patients to come to terms with their disability or physical change. By coming to terms with disability or bodily change we mean people having to re-establish their self-image or the way they see themselves. This type of bodily change is not just a physical problem: it is also a psychological one. In order to understand this clearly we need to take a few moments to look at what a self-image is and how it affects us.

38

MIRROR, MIRROR ON THE WALL . . .

Pantomimes and fairy tales sometimes tell important truths about human beings. As children, perched on the edge of our seats, we wanted to know that the mirror would announce whether or not Snow White was the fairest of them all. As adults who no longer believe in magic mirrors we still ask the question, although in a different way. How we see ourselves and our abilities comes from obtaining feedback from those around us. Instead of magic mirrors we listen to and watch what others express or imply about us. We take in such information and, depending on our previous experiences, use it as feedback to help us to decide who we are, what we are and where and how we fit into society.

To get an idea of how important the concept of self-image is, think of the many different ways in which you can define yourself. You might be a district nurse, a health visitor, a woman, a man, married, single, divorced, a mother, a father, black, white, Asian, English, or any other category you can imagine. In addition, you may regard yourself as beautiful, plain, kind, athletic, and so on. Regardless of what category you place yourself in, the way you see yourself will help to determine what you do and how well you do it. For example, if I see myself as being tone deaf because everyone always tells me I cannot sing, I would be very unlikely to go out and hire the Albert Hall in order to give a concert. On the other hand, if everyone I meet tells me that my watercolour paintings are marvellous and I believe them, I might try to get a gallery to display them for me.

Self-image is not just limited to classifications or activities. It concerns our belief about ourselves as basically good or bad people, outgoing or reserved, friendly or aloof, etc. In short, self-image enters into every category of our daily lives by telling us who and what we are. It is fundamental to our behaviour. It also tells us whether we are fitting into what we believe we are supposed to be. For example, if I believe that a nurse is supposed to be a compassionate, caring person and I classify myself as a nurse, then I should be compassionate and caring. This is fine if I see myself in that way, but it can become a problem if I do not see myself as compassionate and caring and yet still classify myself as a nurse. If I am a nurse but am not what nurses are supposed to be, then how do I fit in? In order to make all of the parts fit, I am going to have to change either the way I see myself, or my idea of what a nurse is, or leave the nursing profession.

Try to imagine then what might happen if who and what you are, and have been for many years, suddenly changes. What would happen if the you with whom you are familiar today becomes someone completely different tomorrow? Especially if what you have become does not fit in with what you think you are *supposed* to be like. Yet this is precisely what happens to patients who suddenly develop disabilities or have to suffer bodily changes.

Which brings us back to the three areas we listed at the beginning of this chapter. In each of these areas the individual's existing idea of what he or she is supposed to be like is threatened. Once these physical changes occur, major adjustments have to take place in the person's self-image.

DIALYSIS PATIENTS

Many patients who find themselves needing dialysis discover it to be a double-edged sword. The very procedure which offers them life and relieves them of the worst effects of their illness also acts as a tie by which that life becomes limited and defined. Dialysis becomes not only their saviour, but also a prison. While it allows them to return to work and to go about their daily routine, it also ties them to a procedure without which they will become ill again and risk death.

How people react to the news that they will be 'tied' to a machine for the foreseeable future will depend on the individual. Some will adjust to that change in their lives better than others. However, certain phases seem common to almost all dialysis users.

Adjusting to dialysis

Current thinking about accepting or getting used to the idea of haemo-dialysis distinguishes three basic stages. The first is generally referred to as the 'honeymoon' stage, and, as the name implies, is seen by the patient as basically good. Hope is high and the patient is feeling much better. It is at this time that most patients are more pleased at their own improvement than upset at the prospect of being dependent on a machine for the rest of their lives. When people have not been able to get out at all, even a little improvement in their ability to get up and around is a welcome change.

The second stage typically comes a few months after the start of dialysis, and is referred to as the 'period of disenchantment'. At this stage people experience a sharp drop in hope and confidence. They feel sad and helpless. These feelings are almost always related to some event within the patient's life, such as an over-ambitious attempt to return to work or resuming an activity such as strenuous housework, sport or a hectic social life. It is also generally at this point that the patient is most likely to experience medical complications.

The third phase is what might be called the 'adaptation' or 'acceptance' phase. This typically occurs between 3 and 12 months after the beginning of the decrease in hopefulness. Patients begin to accept the situation better and to learn ways of living within their more restricted circumstances. On the other hand, it is at this time that dependence on the machine is most likely to become a problem for the patient, since it is now that patients realize how tied they really are and how restricting dialysis can be. At this point some patients become angry about their restricted lifestyle. It is very common for this anger to be directed towards the very people who are most actively trying to help: the nurses in the dialysis unit, or the family. This is difficult for the families or nurses concerned to understand but is, in fact, a perfectly normal reaction to a distressing situation.

Strangely enough, it is just as the acceptance of a new lifestyle begins that most patients appear to require more and more support from their doctors and nurses. The support is often requested in non-medical areas such as in finding a job, a flat, or in improving their relationship with a spouse or other important person. This is believed by some psychologists to be due to the new ways in which many people have to start seeing themselves after dialysis. The additional support is needed because of changes in the patient's self-image. For many it is not a change from 'sick' to 'well yet dependent'; it is more like a change from 'well' to 'well yet dependent'. This often means to the patient that he or she is less capable of managing his or her own affairs than before. Inevitably this is reinforced on every occasion that the patient must undergo treatment.

Limits to the patient's mobility can be exaggerated by a sense of being socially restricted as well. Strict limitations in diet or alcohol intake demanded by dialysis may well not only require a change in eating or drinking habits but also lead to a loss of current friends and social routine. If a patient's main form of relaxation before being taken ill was to go to the local pub and have a few pints with friends, the chances of being able to do so again are not very high. For the nurse who sees dialysis as a life-saving procedure which allows the patient to continue a productive life it may be very difficult to understand the patient's view of it as a restrictive process, costing all those friends and habits which were so familiar and enjoyable. Therefore it may be difficult to understand why someone is so angry and hostile towards the very people who are attempting to help.

Difficulty in adjustment which can lead to anger can also result in distress for the whole family. This is especially likely if the person who is affected is the family bread-winner. If being the bread-winner is no longer possible because of treatment, then it is not easy for that patient to maintain their place in the family structure and much easier to feel a failure.

Before the onset of serious kidney problems, Howard had been a print worker earning a very reasonable wage. When he had to give up work and live on a disability pension he became very grumpy and bad tempered, especially towards his wife Cath, who worked as a barmaid. Even though his disability pension actually brought in more money than her earnings, he felt undermined and superfluous. He told Cath that she was deliberately trying to make a fool of him, and was showing him up in front of his mates. She thought he was being ridiculous, and eventually lost patience with him. Their relationship gradually deteriorated, and when at last he tried to forbid her from continuing work, she decided she had had enough, and packed her bags and left.

Marital problems are not the only area of difficulty. Restrictions such as not being able to go on holiday due to a fixed treatment routine can help generate feelings of responsibility and self-blame within the patient. The nurse may have to help not only the patient but other members of the family to understand the requirements and functions of the treatment. This includes a close and honest look at the problems as well as the advantages of modern dialysis treatment. Sometimes patients will simply decide that it is not worth the effort, and the nurse may well have an important role to play in encouraging patients to be more realistic and less demanding of themselves. When patients *have* to change jobs or lifestyles due to dialysis treatment, it is often the nurse who can provide the support and structure that is needed in the process of developing more appropriate activities and habits. Adopt a problem-solving approach, which should include these stages:

- Sit down with your patient and the patient's spouse. Ask them to talk about those things in life which are most important for them personally and what targets they are now aiming for.
- Ask them what particular problems they are encountering which prevent them from achieving those targets.
- Ask them to list the solutions that might be possible. Emphasizing the fact that you are working on this together, work out a plan for implementing some of those solutions.

- Next time you visit, ask whether any of the proposed solutions worked. If not, try again.

OSTOMY PATIENTS

People who have undergone either colostomies or ileostomies are likely to have some of the same problems as people undergoing dialysis, but they also have some problems that are unique to themselves. Not only are they not functioning as they think they are 'supposed' to, but they also have the problem of possible embarrassment in public. In truth, most ostomy patients are unnoticeable to other people. Unfortunately, when first told of the need for an ostomy, many fear that the required bag will be visible to everyone. They fear that their clothes will not hang right and that anyone passing will be able to pick them out by smell alone. The possibility that there will be a leakage or breakage is a constant fear for many, even years after the operation. Again, as with dialysis patients, there is a concern that they will be seen as less desirable or likeable, especially by the opposite sex, because they are not 'in full working order'.

As very young children we are trained not to soil ourselves. Toilet training is seen as so important that a great deal has been written about it in both psychology and baby-rearing books. Control is often equated with being good, and soiling with being bad. Children often fear that if control is lost and soiling takes place they will risk losing the love and support of those who are most important and close to them, whether they are parents or teachers, and also be ridiculed by their friends. It is understandable then that people who have undergone an operation which has caused them to lose that very control might see the results as threatening, and themselves as being 'bad' or dirty. Because of this, one of the main initial worries of new ostomy patients is the fear of a breakage or leakage. Such a fear can persist in the face of repeated reassurance that it is very unlikely to happen. Even the smallest leak may be exaggerated in the mind of the patient and used to make existing fears greater.

A second fear that many ostomy patients report is their concern about odours. Again this tends to persist in spite of the most insistent denial by those close to the patient.

Jim, a recent ostomy patient, was quite open about his worries. When asked how he dealt with the problem, he said that he seldom went out where there were other people, especially if the meeting was to take place indoors. He always made certain that he was in an open area and that there was a good breeze or air circulation wherever he was inside. These precautions were even more carefully adhered to when he was in the company of women. It took a lot of persuasion and reassurance on the part of the health visitor who was looking after Jim to convince him that such precautions were unnecessary and self-limiting.

Because of such fears, the ostomy patient is very often likely, like Jim, to shy away from social situations and contacts. This has a worsening effect in that there is no way for the person to find out from other people that the fears are in fact unfounded. As the person becomes more and more of a recluse, so fears of other people can develop which isolate the individual even more. The nurse can be a primary contact in breaking this type of cycle, simply by providing plenty of reassurance and accurate information.

The nurse can also be important in another way. Many ostomy patients as well as dialysis patients report that they feel they cannot discuss their problems with others since they fear being embarrassed or being labelled as weak, dirty or strange. Often family members will not go along and attend dialysis treatments or help an ostomy patient with the changing of the bag or cleaning which is necessary. All too commonly the family view the procedure as frightening or dirty too, and this opinion is easily transmitted to the patient. Trying to tell an ostomy patient that there is nothing to fear is difficult when the patient's spouse or family will not touch the bag or even enter the room when replacements are being fitted. As much care needs to be offered to other family members as to the patient. If the nurse can effectively involve the spouse in maintenance procedures, the patient will benefit through being valued as a person, not simply categorized or rejected as a problem.

MASTECTOMY PATIENTS

It is widely known that cancer of the breast is a major killer of young and middle-aged women in the Western world. In helping patients who have cancer of the breast, psychological as well as physical factors are extremely important.

The symbolic importance of the breast

Throughout history, the breast has been the chief symbol of femininity. It has symbolized the maternal capabilities which are both biologically and culturally assigned to women, and has long been seen as the source of nurturance and maternal comfort. Hence women's breasts have been sculpted and painted by many of our greatest artists over the years. It is the breast that feeds the children, thus symbolizing the primary role of women in maintaining all cultures – that of bearing and raising children. Until relatively recently, even within our culture, this was seen by many as the major role for a woman. The ability to give birth and feed babies defined for a young woman who she was and what she was destined to become. Without breasts a woman could not suckle a child and so the child could not grow. The woman without breasts could not fulfil her role and was consequently not seen as desirable. Only relatively recently have these ideas have been successfully challenged on a widespread basis, so that some women at least have been able to develop their lives in other directions as well.

At the same time, however, other social trends re-emphasize the breast. As a result of the advent of many popular magazines and newspapers, an increase in the acceptability of public nudity, and the pressures of modern advertising, women's breasts have become simultaneously less maternal and more obviously sexual. In addition, as bottle feeding has became more popular, so women's breasts are no longer seen as the only source of nourishment for children. So while the nurturing function of breasts may or may not be seen as necessary by many women, their sexual function is probably seen as more important by most women.

The view that many women are deeply concerned about their appearance is supported in part by the amount of money spent each year on cosmetics and in part by the numbers of women who diet in order to achieve the 'ideal' look or body. In our current culture the 'best' female body is young and slim, with two somewhat protuberant breasts. Since this image is held up as the 'ideal' or most desirable, it is very easy for many women to see anything less as diminishing their self-worth and attractiveness.

These then are some of the reasons why the loss of a breast is felt to be so devastating by many women. For some it might mean the loss of purpose in life or the inability to achieve a goal like breast-feeding a child. But for almost all women it is generally seen (at least initially) as a loss of self-worth and desirability, both as an individual and as a sexual partner.

In the case of a radical mastectomy, the loss of the breast usually follows immediately after the diagnosis of active cancer. The woman in such a situation faces impending death, and yet realizes that the only way to avoid it is to take away that which most outwardly denotes her as a woman. The fact that breast cancer kills more women than any other disease, whilst early detection and surgery can often arrest or cure it, points to the magnitude of the decision facing women when they suspect or are told that they have breast cancer which may require a mastectomy.

Let us make it absolutely clear at this point that in no way do we support or wish to perpetuate any idea that equates femininity, a woman's self-worth, or sexuality, with any part of her body or appearance. In fact, it is very much the opposite. To say that the self-worth or sexuality of a woman is dependent merely on her body is a denial of the essence of her personality. Nevertheless, it is remains true that the sense of mutilation, both to the woman and her partner, can be devastating.

Recognizing the nurse's own feelings

How we view our bodies and feel about them does affect our sense of well being, and parts of our body are inextricably linked to our feelings of being a person, even though we must avoid the trap of thinking that this is all there is to a person. The pressures of society have led many women (including nurses) to believe that fewer than two breasts equals less than a whole *person*, when in reality it means less than a whole *body*. Hence female nurses can feel uneasy and somewhat vulnerable when working with mastectomy patients, whilst many male nurses may also become uncomfortable in trying to deal with a situation of which they not only have no direct experience but will never have to face personally. It is difficult for a nurse simultaneously not to succumb to feelings of vulnerability; to be aware of the fact that the breast does not define the person; and at the same time not to lose sight of the fact that the breast is *not* separate from the person. Being aware of all these things at the same time is the most complex psychological issue be faced by nurses working with mastectomy patients.

Marianne was a 26-year-old nurse who was asked to provide follow-up treatment for a 65-year-old mastectomy patient, Mrs Fry. The doctor with whom Marianne worked was exceptionally aware of how sensitive an issue mastectomy often is, and asked Marianne if she had any major reservations about taking it on. Marianne said she would be happy to see the patient. She foresaw no major difficulties and accepted the case.

The first two or three visits went quite well as dressings were changed and Marianne and Mrs Fry discussed the specific details of the surgery and follow-up care. It wasn't until Marianne noticed that Mrs Fry's husband always left the room when dressings were changed that she asked Mrs Fry how things were getting along between them. She was quite surprised by the amount and degree of anger that Mrs Fry suddenly expressed, much of it directed at Marianne. Looking back at the incident later Marianne was also quite surprised at her own reaction and the degree of anger and defensiveness which she had shown in return.

It just so happened that Marianne was on holiday for the next week, so another nurse from Marianne's team took over the care of Mrs Fry for the week. During her holiday Marianne spent some time thinking about the situation. On returning to work she went back to see Mrs Fry. They were both initially uncomfortable, but Marianne was eventually able to explain to Mrs Fry that while she had not undergone what Mrs Fry had, she also felt very vulnerable and that this had, no doubt, played a part in her reaction to Mrs Fry's outburst. They were also able to talk about some of Mrs Fry's fears and concerns. During their discussion Marianne learned that Mrs Fry had refused to allow her husband near her because she was afraid that if he saw her without one of her breasts he would no longer love her. She also found that Mrs Fry refused to leave the house because she was afraid that everyone would know that she had had one of her breasts removed. Even though Marianne tried to convince Mrs Fry that neither of these assumptions was necessarily true, Mrs Fry continued to repeat them, saying that Marianne didn't understand because she was too young and was 'still OK'.

Marianne then spoke to the prosthetics nurse connected to her health team, and arranged for her to visit Mrs Fry at home. Soon Mrs Fry was fitted with a prosthetic breast, and was shown many styles of clothing that were both comfortable and attractive. She was also introduced to a member of a local mastectomy support group and found that she could discuss her problems and fears with someone who had also suffered from cancer in the past. Marianne continued to see Mrs Fry, and soon they discovered that they, too, could talk about many of the worries that they both had. Mrs Fry's husband was finally brought into the discussions. Both Mrs Fry and Marianne were surprised to discover the extent to which he had felt left out and 'discarded' throughout the course of Mrs Fry's illness and recovery. They also learned that as his wife had become more frightened and defensive during her illness he had

tended to withdraw more to give her 'more space', which she interpreted
as a rejection of her, which he interpreted as a rejection of him, and so
on into a vicious circle.

The implication of what we have been saying is that of all the cancers, breast cancer is one of the most threatening on a personal level. Other cancers can be equally or even more disfiguring and distressing. But the nurse working with mastectomy patients has to be even more aware than usual of the psychological factors which are likely to be present. These factors are likely to have a central place in the patient's progress.

THE MANY FACETS OF SELF-IMAGE: HOPE FOR THE FUTURE

A person's self-image is like a finely cut, exquisite diamond. Its beauty is created by the many facets that go toward its make-up. No matter which facet you look into you see a slightly different view of the person. This does not mean that the person is being insincere or 'two-faced' but simply that all people are a combination of many different parts, and that our self-image and identify as people comes from how the different parts of ourselves are combined. But self-image is much less durable than a diamond. As noted in each of our examples, self-image is a surprisingly fragile and sensitive entity, and can be very easily threatened or damaged.

Yet the fact that self-image *is* many-faceted means that helping people to restore their self-image after a loss or problem is that much easier. This is because it is only a part or facet of themselves, and not the whole of themselves, which has been damaged or lost. A nurse can therefore help people to see that if they have lost a limb, or the use of one of their internal organs, then only a part, and not all of them has been lost. This does not mean that the loss or damage should be shrugged off as insignificant. Indeed, the person may well want and need to express a lot of anger and grief connected with the loss, since what has gone may have been a key part of their self-image. If so, they should be encouraged to do so. But it does mean that you can help the person to see that there is more to a person than the sum of the parts of the body. Having a colostomy does not turn you from being a nice, good person into a bad, worthless, unlovable person (as some patients, at least for a while, may think). It turns you into a nice, good person who has had a colostomy. The problem is always thinking in black and white: good and whole, bad and damaged. We are all made up of a combination of parts or facets.

Faced with special problems, it is possible to adapt by discovering new parts of ourselves, such as our capacity to enjoy new, maybe quieter activities, or to help others in the same situation.

The problems of stereotyping

We mentioned earlier in this chapter (and discuss in more detail in Chapter 12) that who we are and what we are is also derived from the groups to which we belong. In this sense, each 'belonging' can be seen as a facet of the diamond of our self-image. Not only do we define ourselves by the groups to which we belong, but we also tend to define other people by the group or groups to which we think they belong. While often giving us some very important information about the people involved, this process of defining people by the groups to which they belong, which is called stereotyping, can create some very difficult problems.

In stereotyping, any negative feelings we have about one particular person within a group tend to be applied unquestioningly to all members of that group. The most obvious example of this occurs with racial or religious prejudice, but the process is not limited to race or religion. It applies to any grouping of which you can think. Because of this, the community nurse may have a lot of difficulty with patients who belong to a group with particular problems if the nurse's prior contact with 'that sort of patient' has been unpleasant or difficult.

Hugh, a community nurse working in a small country town, was referred a brain-damaged patient suffering from multiple injuries after a motor bike accident. During his training Hugh had experienced a similar case, which had frightened him badly because of the extent of the injuries. Before even seeing the patient, Hugh had decided it was a hopeless case, and tried to pass on the referral to someone else. It was only because there was no one else available to take on the case that Hugh eventually went to visit the patient, and found to his surprise that he could actually establish a reasonable relationship with the patient, and that there was quite a lot that he could do to help. In Hugh's case, stereotyping had very nearly worked against the interests of the patient.

The process of stereotyping is not always overcome so easily. According to many organizations for the handicapped or chronically sick, the main problem faced by their members is not the handicap or illness itself but the attitudes of the able-bodied around them. Too often handicap or illness becomes more important than personality. Yet if I happen to have a mastectomy, I do not wish to be known by all those around me as 'the mastectomy', but as a person who has recently had a particular operation. Likewise, the dialysis or ileostomy patient often wishes that other people would see them as people first, and put the handicap or problem second.

Being on the receiving end

The negative consequences of stereotyping do not apply only to patients. They also apply to us, as members of the helping professions. Why is this, and what happens?

People tend to resist change, especially when it is thrust upon them. We often try our best to keep things as we know and like them to be and expend a great deal of energy to ensure that who and what we are today is the same as who and what we were yesterday and will be tomorrow. Consequently, when familiar things change it is often a source of much discomfort. The discomfort produced by change can be made ever worse when it follows the threat of a life-endangering disease or accident. Two fairly normal reactions to change usually follow: either I can try to explain the change by admitting to the change within myself, or can say that it is due to a change in the world around me, which lead very easily into blaming the world around me for all of my troubles. In circular fashion this can lead to stereotyping again.

Following an illness or surgery which has very major effects on person's self-image, it is easy for people to see the medical profession a a stereotyped group, rather than as a collection of specific individual. The mere fact that you are a nurse and one of the health professional may put you in the same 'group' as the doctors who have just performe restrictive or 'mutilating' surgery. Thus, you may be seen as equall responsible for the patient's current difficulties. At the very time you ar trying your hardest to help someone recover from a very difficu operation, you can find yourself the focus of a great deal of anger an hostility.

So, how should you react? The nurse who can listen carefully to wh is being said without just reacting to the anger and accusations can gain great deal of insight into what is really causing the difficulty for th patient. This sounds easier said than done. With support from yo colleagues (who can reassure you that you are not the cruel ar heartless person you may be accused of being), you can often do a l more good for the patient in the long run. But you *do* need that suppo We discuss this further in Chapter 11.

Why you cannot do everything; or, the limits of help

Another facet of self-image that may create difficulties for a community nurse is tied up with the fact that a lot of our sense of who we are comes from the feedback we get from others. The importance that we place upon the feedback and its capacity to influence us tends to be in direct relation to the importance to us of the person giving it. The more important the person is to us, the more important the feedback. For example, if our boss tells us that our work is good, while at the same time a stranger who thinks nursing is a waste of time anyway tells us that our work is bad, we will generally be more likely to pay attention to what our boss says. Likewise, if a nurse says that a patient has not changed and their spouse walks into the room and says how really different the patient has been lately, most people tend to believe their spouse.

As another example, we mentioned that one of the major concerns of people who have had a colostomy is the worry about the odour and the fear of soiling themselves. If the feedback that they get from you as a nurse is that everything is OK and very little, if anything, has changed (which they may find hard to believe anyway), and at the same time their spouse refuses to touch the bag or makes faces and comments about it as they do touch it, then the problem for the nurse is clear.

It is obvious that it is very helpful for the nurse, in almost all situations and especially in those where a person's self-image is in the process of change, to try to involve a spouse and family members in treatment. It is the family who are most likely to help the patient regain or recreate a self-image. So mobilizing the resources of a family in adapting to the change will help the patient's adaptation, too. The more constructively they can approach the new situation, the more likely will the patient be to develop an attitude of positive acceptance, which facilitates recovery.

With everything to gain, the earlier you start this involvement the better chance there is of getting the desired results. Experience has shown that spouses who are left out of preliminary decisions feel isolated, and tend to detach themselves from helping in the patient's treatment. It is then often very difficult, if not impossible, to encourage them back into a supporting role. Attempts to do so may be met with withdrawal on the part of the patient, which leads into that spiral of non-support which we described in the case of Mrs Fry. The sooner the nurse starts to involve the spouse, the better the chance of maintaining the patient's self-image and encouraging overall improvement. Even if you have come in after the fact, the longer you wait, the more difficult it gets. While yesterday may have been the best day to start, today is much better than tomorrow. Try to involve the family members initially in very simple, non-threatening tasks, only gradually increasing the difficulty of what you are asking them to do. At the same time, ask them about their feelings towards their present circumstances. It may be that the reluctance to help the patient stems from feelings of grief, anger or guilt, and until these feelings are expressed in words, they may be expressed in actions – refusing to get involved with the patient. Show that you understand and accept these feelings, and simultaneously demonstrate how help can be given in many small ways.

CONCLUDING REMARKS

In today's society people constantly compare themselves with others and conclude that they are not as good as them. Patients with special problems are even more likely than the rest of us to decide they are 'no good' because some part of them is damaged or missing. Sometimes it requires a lot of moral courage to believe, contrary to what advertisers and film stars seem to imply, that you can be happy and fulfilled without being physically perfect. Yet happiness comes from within, not without. Even if the nurse cannot put back the missing part of the body, or repair the damaged organ, he or she can at least help someone to develop more self-acceptance and tolerance, through being aware of the self-image issues which are inevitably present in the process of recovery or maintenance treatment procedures.

Suggestions for further reading

Nichols, K.A. (1984) *Psychological Care in Physical Illness*. London: Croom Helm.
  Clearly argued and very persuasive, this book points out how health care professionals are in danger of neglecting the emotional and psychological health of many patients by ignoring their feelings about themselves and their illnesses and concentrating only on physical health. Although academic in style it should be required reading for all health workers.

Levitt, P.M. and Guralnick, E.S. (1985) *The Cancer Reference Book: Direct and clear answers to everyone's questions*. London: Harper and Row.
  This book lives up to the promise of its title: it is clear and honest; useful to both nurses and patients.

Williams, C. (1985) *All About Cancer: A practical guide to cancer care*. Chichester: Wiley.
  Outlines what the common cancers are, what diagnosis involves, and what treatment is generally available. It is based on the principle (which we share) that the patient is best dealt with as a whole person. Honestly and straightforwardly written.

Chapter 5

Death and Bereavement

Nurses are perhaps more familiar with death and dying than any other professional group, since there is a tendency for the terminally ill to receive less rather than more care from doctors. So most of the stress and problems involved in caring for the dying fall on the shoulders of nurses. Community nurses are especially involved in helping to care for people for whom there is no need to stay in hospital and who have chosen to spend the rest of their life at home. Additionally, community nurses are often the people involved in offering counselling and support for the bereaved relatives during the dying process and after a death has occurred.

We start this chapter with the feelings and anxieties that often occur when facing death, and the reactions of relatives to death. Then we consider the role of the nurse in helping the family to cope with the death and the feelings nurses themselves are likely to have when working in this emotionally charged area.

FACING DEATH

Statistics show that nowadays most of us are likely to die of heart or respiratory disease, or cancer. The chances are that we will die in some sort of institution, a hospital, hospice or home for the elderly, rather than in our own homes. Although accidents and violent deaths do occur, these are relatively less frequent than deaths that follow a period of illness.

Surveys have shown that most people do in fact know that they are dying despite the belief of many doctors and nurses that they do not know. Indeed, although medical opinion is mixed about whether the dying person should be told outright that their condition is fatal, most dying people do realize sooner or later that they are unlikely to recover. Furthermore, they want to be able to talk about it. Research has clearly shown that if people know that they are dying, not only do they have the opportunity to arrange their affairs in preparation for their deaths, but they can also deal with 'unfinished business', like making peace with estranged family members, or carrying out some life-long and cherished ambition, and saying goodbye appropriately to loved ones.

The question of whether or not to tell dying patients that they are dying is a vexed one. Many doctors and surgeons have a very straightforward policy that all of their patients should be told of impending death, but the only person who is allowed to tell the patient is the doctor. This puts the attending nurse in a very difficult position, especially if a good, trusting relationship has grown up between nurse and patient. At some point the patient who suspects that something is not quite right may well turn to the nurse and ask quite directly: 'Am I dying, nurse?'. Although some nurses are at this point obliged by the policies laid down in their particular practice to say nothing and to persuade the patient to ask the doctor, some nurses may well take the law into their own hands and feel that it is in the patient's interests that he or she be told. These nurses, and nurses in practices where openness is the policy anyway, have to answer the difficult question.

Giving bad news is not easy. However, most people find uncertainty worse than actual facts. It is perhaps comforting to know that most patients will not ask questions about dying unless they have a pretty shrewd suspicion that they are terminally ill. In addition, the nurse will probably find through experience that a patient will not be able to 'hear' an answer which is too threatening. If patients are not able to cope with what is being said they will often appear to misunderstand the significance of what is being conveyed. However, there are some patients who are not helped by being given more information, and nurses need to become skilled in being able to distinguish this minority of patients, who do not want to learn the worst, from the majority. We discuss this further in Chapter 10.

Patients are often braver about this topic than nurses and doctors. Staff will mistakenly continue not to inform patients for fear of the patient 'falling to pieces'. A sort of pretence then develops, when neither side is telling the truth, although somehow both sides know what is going on. In most cases, an honest, straightforward but very supportive conversation about the future is best at this point. This does not mean to say that it will be easy for either the nurse or the patient. But at least no one will be living a lie or dying unprepared. Giving difficult news is a skill that can be learned.

Most people die when they are over the age of 65, although of course tragic deaths in younger people or even children do take place, and are perhaps more shocking precisely because they are unexpected and unusual. The process of dying is an unfamiliar one for most people. The majority of deaths do take place in institutions of some sort, and death is not an easy thing to talk about. A proper fear of the unknown is almost always present when facing either our own deaths or those of our loved ones. In helping dying patients, find out what they know about their condition, and also what they know about the business of dying. It is only then that the nurse can reach into the distress that is felt. Understanding the fear of pain as distinct from the fear of death may also be helpful. The possibility of pain is more difficult for many people to contemplate than the prospect of death.

Why is dying so distressing?

The prospect of dying is one of life's most stressful and anxiety-provoking experiences, not only because no one really knows what death is like but because people are afraid of the loneliness of death. These two aspects of death, not knowing what is going to happen and fearing being alone, seem to be central to the distress of dying.

Anxiety

Not knowing what is going to happen is a cause of anxiety at all times, but is especially acute in the process of dying. Between a quarter and a half of all terminally ill people report themselves to be anxious and have physical symptoms of stress (described further in Chapter 10). These symptoms include pounding of the heart, loss of appetite, feelings of faintness and breathlessness. All of these may also be present as symptoms of the terminal illness itself. Younger people are more often worried about possible pain and also the impact that their death will have on others; older people are more likely to be anxious about becoming dependent on others and about losing bladder and bowel control. Young children are usually worried about being abandoned by their parents or separated from them. They are more anxious about being in hospital, away from Mum and Dad, than about dying itself. Older children's anxieties are more like those of young adults, centring on pain and loss.

As we would expect, not all people feel the same way or have the same worries. Some people become more anxious as their death approaches, whilst others become calmer and more accepting. There are no general rules, except that a person will probably approach their death in the same way as they approach the rest of their life. That is, someone who has always been in control of everything during their life may find it more difficult to accept dying, which is beyond their control, than someone who has always been more easygoing. Religious views are also important here. Someone who has always been very confident that this life is simply a stepping-stone to a happier and blissful after-life may find death easier to contemplate than someone who has put a lot of emphasis on achieving things in this life and does not believe in a God. Therefore, in order to understand how someone is likely to face death we need to know about their beliefs and attitudes, especially when these come from a different culture.

An example of the way in which personality can affect dying can be seen in the case of Bob. Bob was a very active trade union official, organizing meetings, running courses for activists, and negotiating successfully with high-level management. His diary was always full, and he rarely had a day at work in which nothing was planned. His home-life was as well organized at his work life: weekends were scheduled and organized to enable him and his wife to fit in their wide range of interests and hobbies. Above all, Bob prized being in control of all of his activities, and resented it whenever something unexpected happened to throw his plans out of order. When he suffered a series of coronaries at the age of 56 he was rushed into hospital, where he stayed until he died several weeks later. The last few weeks of Bob's life were very difficult ones for him, as he was unable to take control of the situation he found himself in. His body was in control, not him. This made him very anxious indeed, and he tried to fight what was happening. This of course just made things worse, as anxiety makes people physically tense, and we know that this increases pain, breathlessness and blood pressure.

Loneliness

The second distressing aspect of dying is the loneliness associated with it. Most people do not know what to say to a dying person and so tend to avoid the terminally ill or offer unrealistic hope. In consequence the dying are often very lonely and feel they cannot make themselves understood. Studies of nurses in hospital have shown that nurses will actually avoid going near the bed of a terminally ill patient and make a detour for fear of getting involved in conversation. This is understandable if the nurse has not had much training in how to talk to the dying patient, and if the ward is a busy one. It happens in the community, too. Perhaps the patient who is dying in very upsetting circumstances is the one who somehow does not get as many visits as another patient. It is professionally stressful to share isolation, especially without considerable back-up and support. This support is not always available to the professional, so that the dying person may in turn be very lonely just when someone is most needed.

We also know that people who are lonely are actually *more* likely to die than those surrounded by family and friends. Men and women are social creatures, whose lives are given meaning through relationships with others. Loneliness can actually contribute to illness and death. We know, for example, that someone's death is often followed very quickly by the death of their spouse.

Some patients will want company less than others, and the need for communication varies at different times in the process of dying. As death approaches the need for social conversation usually becomes less, whilst the need simply to have someone around increases. Dying people often just need someone to hold their hand. In the absence of a spouse or family, a nurse or doctor who will not abandon them to the process of dying alone is of immense human value.

Coming to terms with dying

Although not everyone faces death in the same way there do seem to be recognizable stages or states which most dying people experience. Although not everyone goes through each stage, most people experience at least one or two of these stages and also pass back and forth between the stages many times. If someone does not go through a particular stage it does not mean there is anything abnormal or wrong. It simply means that different people have different needs, as well as their own unique ways of expressing themselves. In no way should a nurse who is trying to help a patient come to terms with approaching death attempt to persuade a patient to go through stages which are not appropriate.

One of the best-known writers on the subject of dying is Elisabeth Kübler-Ross, who wrote a best-selling book in 1969 called *On Death and Dying*. Since then, nurses and others working with the dying have used her ideas to help dying patients with skill and sensitivity. Elisabeth Kübler-Ross suggested that there are five basic stages which most people go through when they face death. We list them here, and you will notice how these stages could apply equally well to other kinds of loss, such as divorce or becoming unemployed. If you yourself have at any time had to deal with one of these problems, you will probably remember some of these reactions.

Stage 1: Denial of death

The first reaction to bad news is often to deny it. 'It couldn't happen to me', or 'They will find a cure', or 'A miracle will happen' are all typical responses. The patient will ignore what he or she does not want to know, or assume that someone, somewhere has made a mistake. Doctors and nurses may go along with this denial, with the insistence that the patient should not give up hope. While it is, of course, important that the patient should not become hopeless, professional denial of the seriousness of the illness does not help the patient to come to terms with it, either. Colluding to avoid the inevitable is more damaging than the painful business of dealing with death. A few patients may cling to the belief that they are not dying, right until the end, although this is quite rare. In fact, Elisabeth Kübler-Ross only found 4 out of 500 patients who denied the fact that they were dying right until the moment of death.

Stage 2: Rage

When it no longer becomes possible to deny the fact of dying, the patient may start to express anger and bitterness about the situation. The typical cry at this stage is 'Why me?'. Patients may declare their anger and resentment to anyone around them, such as spouse, nurses, doctors, or God. This can be distressing for families, especially when they too feel angry and upset by the news and have to take the brunt of the hostility. It is important for those who are dealing with the dying person to realize that the anger and hostility being expressed are not directed at them 'personally', but are in fact an expression of distress.

Bob, the trade union official, became rather abusive towards the nurses in the intensive care unit to which he was admitted, as he tried to deny the fact that he was no longer in total control of his life. It was not the nurses that he was really angry with, but the failure of his own method of coping, which had otherwise stood him in such good stead throughout his life.

Stage 3: Bargaining

Once the rage and anger has diminished, patients may attempt to do something constructive about their situation, like trying to strike a bargain with fate, or God, to allow them time to finish a particular task, or to delay the death until after an especially important event. In return for a few more weeks of life, patients will promise to be especially 'good' or do something in exchange. In fact, these 'bargains' often seem to be quite effective, in that people will sometimes die after their birthdays, after Christmas, or following some special event like the wedding of a favourite grandchild.

Mrs Sullivan was suffering from severe kidney problems and had been told that there was only a limited amount of time left before the kidneys failed completely. Her grand-daughter Suzie was expecting a child and it was only after the birth had been announced that Mrs Sullivan 'allowed' herself to die.

Stage 4: Depression

The feelings of sadness and impending loss are acutely experienced by the dying person after the stages of denial, rage and bargaining. Life seems pointless and extremely sad. Depression as a reaction at other points of life tends to happen in one of three situations:

- following some devastating loss, usually of a significant and loved person
- when a person feels that he or she cannot control what happens any more
- when the things that previously brought happiness are no longer present.

All these three feelings are common in dying people. If they are physically very sick, they may no longer be able to do the things that previously brought them pleasure, like taking the dog for a walk, going out for a drink or cuddling their children. Also, like Bob, they may no longer be able to do anything about their lives, and therefore feel helpless, hopeless and not in control. They will also be aware of the impending loss of their family and friends.

Perhaps the most distressing aspect of dying is the loneliness that often accompanies the process. It is not always the case that dying people are avoided by others, but rather that they cut themselves off.

The diagnosis of an extremely malignant carcinoma of the breast led Linda to withdraw almost completely from her husband. She spent most of her days wrapped up in a blanket, staring out into the garden, and refusing invitations from friends and family to spend time with them. She gradually stopped eating, and lost more weight than would have been expected from her illness. She spurned all attempts made by Mike, her husband, to talk and share the time they had left together in doing things that they both used to enjoy. The sensitive observation by a visiting community nurse that Linda was severely depressed led to a referral to a psychiatrist, who was then able to talk to Linda and prescribe some antidepressant medication. When the depression lifted somewhat Linda was able to tell Mike how lonely she had felt despite his efforts. She had in fact been trying to distance herself from him, in order to reduce the pain that she knew he must be feeling. As a result, both of them had felt utterly miserable and were consequently unable to help one another. After the depression lifted, and Mike understood what had been going on, they were able to draw together again for the last few weeks of Linda's life. She eventually died with Mike's arms around her.

Not all patients who are dying become as severely depressed as Linda, though most will go through a stage of mourning and grief for the impending loss. They will feel regret for all of the things that they should have done and all of the things they wasted time on. A successful businessman may regret the time that he spent with colleagues rather than with his children, or there may simply be grief for the people and things that will soon no longer be. A musician may regret the loss of her ability to play again with her orchestra, or a bus driver the companionship of the bus crews. A mother may mourn the impending loss of her whole family and grieve at the knowledge of how her death will affect them. This stage is labelled by Elisabeth Kübler-Ross as 'preparatory grief', and it allows the person to get ready to die and say goodbye. Because there is a lot of thinking and reviewing going on inside, dying people often seem to withdraw from friends and family at this point. It is not that they do not care any more, but rather that they are working at separating themselves from all that they know and love.

Stage 5: Acceptance

This is the final stage in the dying process, although not all terminally ill people will accept the coming of death, and many will cling very tenaciously to life. For accident victims and young people, this stage is much less likely to occur, as the loss of their lives when others of their age still have years of life stretching ahead all seems so unfair. But for some people at least this is the point at which death becomes an inevitable and not unwelcome conclusion to life. This is especially likely after many weeks or months of struggling with a terminal illness. Modern methods of pain control leave many patients relatively free of pain in the last few weeks of life, although they may be emotionally and physically worn out. Most people do not die suddenly, but slip gradually into unconsciousness. At this point, patients may not be frightened or unwilling to die, but will instead feel very weary, though some may also be in pain and look to death for relief of suffering.

It is at this stage that a person may, if not in too much physical pain, be able to experience the peace and tranquillity that comes with knowing that you have done all you could have done, and have said your goodbyes. The dying person may be able then to live the last period of life with contentment, and enjoy the pleasures of every day, such as flowers, sunsets and the love of friends and relatives. There is no longer any need to deny death and to cling to future plans which can never be fulfilled.

Not all dying patients go through all of these stages, and many go back and forth through them many times. Nurses should not expect their patients to be at any one stage at any one time. Some people approach death by gradually withdrawing from life and preparing for the event with care and forethought. Such people are likely to have drawn up their wills, made plans for dependents and so forth. Others are so busily involved in life that their death appears as an interruption, rather than a planned-for event. Neither approach is 'right' or 'wrong'. It cannot be overstressed that people cope with the fact of death in their own way. Hence, community nurses have to be sensitive to the particular way in which each individual patient chooses to face death, and help that person cope most effectively, whatever the strategy chosen.

Dying children

Maybe the most distressing job for a nurse is to have to care for a dying child. The cruelty of life seems to be most obvious when the person who is facing death is an innocent child who has so much life to lose. The nurse often has to cope with the acute distress of the child's parents, as well as a personal sense of injustice and grief. Children themselves may in fact feel less grief than adults. We know that children under the age of five or six have no very clear idea of the finality of death, and their anxieties are mostly about being separated from their families. On the other hand, children are very good at picking up the signals that others are worried, and will actually do what they can to comfort their parents or nurses. Children between the ages of six and 10 or so become more anxious about possible pain, although their worries about being parted from their families are still more important. Some children may have a reasonably clear picture of the process of dying at this stage, and may well be more matter-of-fact about it than the adults around them.

Danny, a child suffering from muscular dystrophy, asked his mother why she was giving him the model train he had asked for as a Christmas present in the middle of September. When she refused to say why, he said to her in quite a normal voice, 'It's because I might not be here for Christmas, isn't it Mummy?'. In some ways, Danny was more willing to face the impending tragedy than his mother.

Later in this chapter and in Chapter 11, we talk about the kinds of feelings that nurses are likely to experience when facing the deaths of patients to whom they are close. It is enough for the moment to say that such feelings are likely to be particularly acute when the dying person is a child. Nurses working in this area should be especially careful to give themselves and their colleagues plenty of support and back-up of a practical and an emotional kind. Only then will nurses be able to give the parents of a dying child the kind of help which they may desperately need.

BEREAVEMENT

Much of the day-to-day work of nurses in the community is, of course, not with the patient but with the relatives and family of the patient. Nowhere is this work more crucial than with the family of someone who has just died. Bereavement counselling is a regular part of the work of the community nurse, who can contribute a great deal to lessening the distress felt by very unhappy people at a difficult time in their lives.

Just as the dying are all different, and face their own deaths in their own unique way, so too the process of bereavement is different for each family. Nevertheless, there are some typical patterns or phases which have been observed by people who have worked extensively with the bereaved, though it is crucial to realize that recovery from bereavement is complicated and takes very different forms for different people. In addition, the process of grieving takes longer for some than for others.

What does bereavement mean?

Bereavement is generally understood to be the loss by death of someone whose absence is strongly felt. It is perhaps the most devastating and severe life trauma. Following bereavement people are much more likely to become ill themselves, or even die. This is especially so for widowers within the first six months of the death of their wives, and such deaths are often caused by diseases which are made worse by stress and lack of self-care. Widows, too, often die within two years of the death of their husband.

As the people who are hit hardest by death are parents and spouses, this part of the chapter discusses bereavement as it applies to those who have lost either a child or a spouse. This does not mean that other losses are insignificant, but that we are going to limit the discussion to what are normally the most devastating bereavements.

The usual response to bereavement is grief and mourning. The person feels a great sense of loss and a tearing away of a part of themselves. Indeed, the bereaved *have* lost a part of themselves: that part which lived through the relationship with the now dead person. For example, if my child should die, I should lose the part of me which is my son's parent: part of *me* would be dead, too. Or if my spouse should die, I would lose the part of myself that only really exists when we are together. In addition, of course, I may also lose some very important practical things, like some of my income, and some of my social life. I will also lose my identity as a 'married person', and become a 'widow' or 'widower'.

Another way of looking at bereavement is to see it as a loss of some very important attachment or link. It has been suggested by two psychiatrists, John Bowlby and Colin Murray Parkes, that normal people react to bereavement rather as children or young animals react when they are separated from their mothers. That is, the bereaved person will cry out, search for the lost person, resent anybody who seems to prevent them from keeping the memory alive, and so on. The aim of the bereaved at this point is reunion with the dead.

Phases of recovery from bereavement

You may notice as you read through this account of the stages of bereavement how similar it is to the account that we gave of the stages of adjustment to death. In many ways they are similar processes, as in both cases the person has to come to terms with very unwelcome major changes.

The first reaction to bereavement is shock. The bereaved spouse or parent at first refuses to believe the truth, especially if the death was unexpected. At this point people may appear calm and numb. If they have always had difficulty in talking about their feelings they will find it particularly hard to cry. To other people the bereaved individual may appear to be almost in a daze. The funeral is often held during this period and the person is congratulated 'for taking it all so well'.

The second phase develops as the truth of the loss sinks in. Now the parent or spouse may simultaneously feel anger and grief. They may express rage at themselves, God or the health service for not having prevented the death. They may appear to 'search' for the dead person, as suggested by Colin Murray Parkes. At the same time they will feel intensely sad. They will be preoccupied by thoughts and memories of the dead person. This is made worse by all of the reminders of the absence. A mother will keep finding her little daughter's toys; a husband will have to sit and look at the empty armchair opposite him in the evenings. The house will appear to be very empty and quiet. Sometimes the bereaved person will report having seen the dead person in a crowd of faces, or perhaps in dreams. This usually happens because the bereaved person is spending so long thinking about the dead one that anything which is unclear or unfamiliar (like a shadow, a dream or a stranger's face) can be interpreted as being the dead person. In sum, the parent or spouse may feel utterly lost, not knowing how to go on living. Indeed, they have not yet learned any way of adjusting to the loss, or living without the dead one.

The period of intense grief typically lasts for about four to 10 weeks. The next phase of bereavement is the process of recovery. Gradually the bereaved learn to fill the space that has been left by the dead person. That is, they develop new ways of behaving, thinking and feeling which are not totally centred on the dead person and take account of the person's absence. This does not mean that the dead person has been forgotten, but that thoughts stop being concentrated only upon the dead person, initially for brief periods, but then for longer stretches of time. Occasionally there may even be feelings of hope about the future. Practical changes may have to be made. For example, the widow may decide to move to live near her children, or the bereaved parent may give away the child's clothes and toys to charity. But it is important that changes are not made too suddenly. Any attempt to 'replace' the dead one, for example by marrying again, or having another child, should not be made too quickly. Otherwise the grieving process will not have been completed, and the person will be less able to develop new and healthy relationships in the long run.

Some people seem to be better able to cope with bereavement than others. Colin Murray Parkes has looked at married people who make a successful recovery from bereavement. He found that widows and widowers who were fairly independent in their marriages did better, and so did people who were able to face both the good and bad things about their dead spouse. People who appeared to be 'at risk' included those who were bereaved as a result of a sudden unexpected death, and those who felt a lot of anger, guilt, despair and yearning. Women also seem to have a harder time than men in adjusting to the death.

What does this imply for bereavement counselling?

Just as different patients cope with dying in different ways, so bereaved people have their own unique ways of coping with the loss of their loved ones. The community nurse must assess each patient and take into account not only the length of time since the death but also the particular personality of the bereaved person. It would be quite wrong to impose onto one bereaved wife the ways of coping found helpful by another. For one person, the opportunity to have a good laugh about old times may well be just what is needed, while another may just want to cry. Most people do, however, want to be able to talk about the dead person at some time or another. The process of talking seems to assist the bereaved one to adjust to the loss.

A mistake that is commonly made by nurses and others when engaged in bereavement counselling is to think that getting the bereaved person to cry is the most important thing. Lack of crying does not in itself mean that the patient is denying grief, as there are lots of different ways of grieving. While the expression of grief is important at some stage in coming to terms with the loss, it should not be seen as the goal of counselling. The nurse has, therefore, to enquire very gently about the progress of the grieving process before starting to encourage any particular topic of conversation. Often, people are resolving the grieving process in their own way, and encouraging another form of the expression of grief is actually not productive, and may take the person back to an earlier phase.

The following steps are involved in effective bereavement counselling, although they do not need to be taken in this order.

- First, the nurse can help the parent or spouse to acknowledge the loss by talking about it. In this way the bereaved person begins the business of making sense out of a world without the dead person.

- Second, the nurse can be there as a form of emotional support as needed. For a limited time the bereaved person can be dependent on the nurse as someone to confide in and provide support.
- Third, the nurse can help by listening to and accepting any feelings of guilt or self-reproach that the parent or spouse may have. Often the bereaved person may recall arguments which were not resolved, or harsh words which were said, or worse, may blame themselves in some way for the death.
- Fourth, the nurse should encourage the gradual reinvolvement of the bereaved person in social life. Of course, this has to be done at the person's own pace and with a lot of support.

Cindy's daughter was tragically killed while on a shopping errand for her mother, and although Cindy had always done her best to teach her daughter good road sense the little girl had run out in front of a speeding car when she saw a friend across the road. Cindy found it very hard to forgive herself for sending the little girl out on that fatal errand. The nurse's role here was to listen and accept the 'confessions' and help Cindy to see them in perspective.

In brief, the role of the nurse in counselling a bereaved person is to offer acceptance, understanding of the suffering and encouragement. A very clear description of how the bereavement counsellor might act has been provided by Colin Murray Parkes:

Among the most important gifts a therapist can make to a client is respectful interest . . . by drawing on (the) therapist's understanding of their suffering, the bereaved may gain compassion and forgiveness towards themselves. Beyond this, although they will not expect it, they may discover respect for their abilities to come through, and from this respect may gain the further confidence they will need to fully inhabit the lives that lie ahead of them (Murray Parkes and Weiss (1983), pp. 249–250).

A WORD ABOUT NURSES AND DEATH

The final part of this chapter concerns the nurse and death: both the nurse's reaction to patients' deaths, and nurses' thoughts about their own deaths. Working with dying people is a very stressful aspect of the nurse's job, as is bereavement counselling. Small wonder then that working with the dying and bereaved is linked with high levels of stress in nurses. This is especially true for those working with children, cancer patients, and in intensive care units.

Working with the dying is not only distressing because of the feelings of compassion and shared loss which the nurse may feel for the family, but also because it makes nurses think about their own deaths. Most people avoid thinking about this topic, and assume that death will come at some unspecified time in the hazy future. In fact, people generally repress thoughts about their own death and for most people this is probably a reasonably healthy thing to do. But nurses who work with the dying or bereaved are less able to forget about death. Watching people die on a regular basis, or sharing the grief of bereaved families, is bound to make you, as a sensitive, caring person, think about the meaning of death to you. Some hospitals arrange special training for nurses to think and talk through their own feelings about death, but this is still quite rare. Some nurses may find that their own religious beliefs are a help. But for others, religious beliefs may even be challenged by the apparent cruelty of death. They may feel unsure about whether or not there is an after-life, or even whether they want to believe in a God who can sometimes seem so uncaring. You may yourself have wondered how and when you will die, and whether life has any deeper meaning.

There are no easy answers to any of these questions, whether or not you are religious. But in the face of this uncertainty, we do as professionals need to share our feelings and fears with one another. Somehow, most of us do go on living and find some meaning in doing everyday things to the best of our abilities. A preoccupation with death is not productive, because life is short and perhaps the only thing we can do, in the end, is to get on with it. A very wise and experienced writer and doctor named Victor Frankl, who survived a number of dreadful years in German concentration camps during World War II, and had to witness not only the deaths of all of his family and friends, but also the destruction of his home and work, wrote *The Will to Meaning*. He describes how human beings strive to find meaning in something, even in the face of the most dreadful horror. This meaning need not be religion, but can be some political ideal, an ambition, art, or, simply, a belief in human love. In the end, this belief will often transcend the pain of facing death.

If you can tolerate the stresses and unique strains created by professional involvement with dying patients and their families, you may find that it is highly rewarding. We have concentrated here on the problems and difficulties involved in this type of work. But do not forget that there is also a profound satisfaction to be gained from helping people to face this most taxing of life's challenges with dignity and humanity.

Suggestions for further reading

Bond, S. (1982) Communications in cancer nursing. In M.C. Cahoon (ed.) *Recent Advances in Cancer Nursing, 3*. London: Churchill Livingstone.
A nurse with extensive experience with cancer sufferers, Senga Bond here outlines her belief that communication is a key skill in working with cancer patients. She emphasizes the need to communicate with both patients and their families, honestly and sympathetically.

Frankl, V. (1971) *The Will to Meaning*. London: Souvenir Press.
This book outlines Frankl's optimistic message that the discovery of some purpose or meaning in life is the most important goal for us all, whether we are facing death now or at some unspecified point in the future. It could be of help to anyone who is working with dying patients.

Kübler-Ross, E. (1969) *On Death and Dying*. New York: Macmillan.
This is Elisabeth Kübler-Ross' best-known book, which outlines her experiences over many years of working with dying patients. It is both inspiring and sensible in its approach.

Parkes, C. Murray (1975) *Bereavement: Studies of grief in adult life*. Harmondsworth: Penguin.
Nurses carrying out bereavement counselling can get an enormous amount of help from this book, which also discusses the effects of separation and loss in other areas of life.

Stedeford, A. (1984) *Facing Death: Patients, families and professionals*, London: Heinemann.
This book is an account of interviews with couples where one partner is dying. It is both compassionate and sensible, and talks about bereavement as well as the process of dying. Enormously helpful for nurses wanting to know what patients and their relatives are likely to be feeling when facing death.

Chapter 6

Families in the Real World: The Problems of Disruption

The past few centuries have seen many changes in science, communication, medical care and transportation, to name but some of the major influences on our lives. The basic family structure has also seen its share of changes. Divorce rates are increasing annually, and children, parents, and grandparents are less likely to be all living together in the same house. The number of children born to each family is dropping too. Meanwhile members of many families are frequently having to go farther from home in order to find work or to go to school, and temporary or even permanent separations are commonplace.

Because of changes like this, there is an ever-increasing gap between what we actually experience and what we may think of as the 'perfect' family. We are constantly exposed by the media not only to what is 'real', but also to what advertisers and writers (and our own romantic view of the past) would like us to believe is real. This changing family structure can lead to a number of problems, including the idea that what most of us have is not 'normal' and that if only we could force things back to how we imagine they were in the past all would be well.

But these ideas are based on ignorance of what really went on in the past, as well as a lack of knowledge of what actually goes on in most families today. Like it or not, things do change, in the family as elsewhere. So what is happening in families nowadays?

CHANGES AND DISRUPTIONS IN FAMILY STRUCTURE

Firstly, a general point about all families. As people enter and leave the family the other members must redefine their own roles. This means that family members have to adjust to the new relationships and find new ways of behaving with each other. This process is not always a smooth one. For example, when a new baby is born, the existing children have to adjust to the presence of the newcomer. This can sometimes be painful and result in feelings of jealousy and resentment. Such feelings are part of a process of adjustment. If they resolve as more adjustments are made, well and good. If they persist, specific help may be required.

Secondly, some very new things are happening to the family which mean that entirely new patterns of behaviour have to be developed. Traditional roles for men and women are changing fast, which can lead to considerable strain. As we have already noted, the divorce rate is increasing, and step-parenting is becoming almost commonplace. Since community nurses are required to enter the homes of their patients it is no wonder that they often find themselves dealing with families who are under strain because of the changes that are imposed upon the family unit. Such changes can be extremely disruptive.

However, a change does not have to be unexpected or even imposed from outside to be a disruption. Even those changes that are considered and planned for in advance can create a disruption in a home. Marriages, deaths following a long illness, and children going off to college are examples of such changes. But at least these changes are experienced as being a 'normal' part of family development. Changes of this sort will not therefore be the subject of this chapter. Rather, we are concerned here with families where the disruption is painful or unproductive.

WHAT IS A DISRUPTED FAMILY?

Perhaps as a result of the influence of the mass media combined with our own sense of what would be ideal or perfect, when we think of a family, we think of a very traditional group consisting of a father, mother and two or more children. As any nurse who has been working for even a short period of time is aware, however, not all families are like this. Disrupted families are families in which there *was* a traditional family structure at one time in the past, but for some reason it has now changed. Perhaps one or more of the family members have now left, or else remain but are no longer a contributing part of the family.

There are some similarities between non-traditional families and those which are disrupted. Examples of non-traditional families are single-parent families, where the parent chooses to remain single, and communal families, where people live in groups, usually as friends, and often share tasks such as child care, food preparation and home maintenance.

In both these settings, disruption may be experienced, but it is not necessarily part of such alternative families. Many single parent families function well, and the family members are both happy and well adjusted. Studies of the kibbutzim in Israel have also shown that communal families may provide as much involvement and stability as any traditional family structure. Therefore, the concern of this chapter is not with these and other alternatives to the traditional family, but with those families where the traditional structure of mother, father and child(ren) has been disrupted in a way that is not experienced by the members as either beneficial or happy.

WHAT KINDS OF DISRUPTION ARE THERE?

Disruption can happen in any of five ways. The first is that the family remains together and one or more of the family members just 'tunes out' and ceases to be effective. This person then shares no more than just a very superficial interest in the family as a unit and is only interested in personal concerns, becoming isolated within the family. The person may still be there physically, but his or her emotional concerns and interests lie elsewhere.

The second sort of disruption happens when one or more of the family members is removed from the family with an intention to return at some future date. This may happen because of the demands of work, as with military families, where one member, generally the father, may be sent away for a period of months or years. Or it may happen by law, as when one of the members is sent to prison for a period of time. It may also occur with families where a child is removed from the family due to an extended illness or placement in a foster home. In any of these cases the family is severly disrupted, although the intention of all concerned is to go back to the way things were before the disruption happened.

The third situation in which a family might find itself disrupted is when one or more of its members is removed from the family and has no intention of ever returning. In some cases the split will be complete, whilst in others some level of involvement will still be maintained. This occurs in cases of divorce, and may involve not only the loss of one family member such as the father, but increasingly often may involve the separation of brothers and/or sisters when children are divided between their divorcing parents. If this occurs the family members often continue to stay in some kind of contact with each other, through visits or meetings but the level of involvement in the family as a whole is changed.

The fourth and fifth groups consist of families where one or more members is removed, but either cannot or do not wish to remain in touch. This can happen through death, or when there is a runaway child or an abandoning parent. While there are many similarities between the death of a family member and loss through abandonment or running away, there are also many differences. In most cases a death is seen as final and as having had some specific cause such as an accident or a terminal illness, whereas the loss of someone through their own decision to leave is often fraught with uncertainties and unanswered questions. In many cases this can be at least as painful as death to the remaining person(s), with feelings much more protracted.

Although in many ways these five groups are similar, each of them creates distinct problems for the family and, in consequence, for any nurse who is working them. We will take them one at a time and look at each individually.

Disruption through 'tuning out'

It is not uncommon in real life for family members to have stopped communicating with each other. Conversation which, on the surface, is like the conversations held by artificial families on television, is in fact replaced by superficial exchanges or even by the television itself. Individual members drift apart, and find themselves isolated within the very family structure that is 'supposed' to provide them with comfort and support. Unfortunately, those who 'tune out' are the least likely to say, or be able to say, why they have done so. The most important thing for the nurse to be able to recognize is that the 'tuning out' person has removed himself or herself from the family and that this can make considerable difficulties for the rest of the family. Since the tuning-out person physically remains in the family, he or she can be easily overlooked when trying to discover what is going on within the family.

Michael was always seen as a problem and at seven years old always seemed to be sick. His father was a professional person who made enough money to support his family and to give them many extras, like their recent holiday abroad and all of the expensive toys he had just bought for Michael. He was considered to be loving and caring by all who knew him. In fact he was personally and emotionally detached from the family.

Michael had been referred to the community nursing service following an unusually long recovery from an appendicectomy. Whilst on an assessment visit, Michael's nurse became aware that Michael had very little to say about his father. Since the nurse knew that Michael's father was living at home there seemed to be no reason why he was not included when Michael talked about his family. By bringing the subject up with Michael's mother, the nurse discovered that his father worked well into the evening almost every night, and seldom if ever was home for an entire weekend. As they talked more and more about the situation, Michael's mother admitted that she had been 'on edge' for quite a while and that while Michael's father was 'perfect' he seldom talked to them even when he was at home, leaving Michael and his mother to deal themselves with their day-to-day problems.

Following some encouragement from the nurse, Michael's mother finally convinced her husband that they should seek marriage guidance. As the marriage guidance progressed, Michael recovered quickly, his mother was less edgy, and his father gradually became a more active member of the family, starting to play with Michael again instead of just buying him presents.

Disruption through separation

As society continues to become more and more mobile the difficulty of maintaining strong family ties increases. A number of years ago it was quite common to have three or four generations living together within the same house. Now we find situations in which even husbands and wives are being separated for occupational reasons. This has happened lately not just in jobs which involve lots of travel, such as the military, but also amongst the more stable occupations like the construction trade and upper management in multinational industries. Often, as shown recently in the popular television series *Auf Wiedersehen, Pet*, husbands may even be required to travel to foreign countries to find work to support their families remaining behind.

In contrast to circumstances where there is divorce or death, these people typically do not wish to end their relationship. They try to find ways to continue their relationship with its host of special problems. Whenever one partner wants to ask something of the other, either an expensive phone call is required or several days of waiting before getting an answer. In a culture where we expect a reasonably quick response to questions, such a delay can be extremely frustrating.

Jan and David had been married for five years and had a three-year-old daughter named Stephanie, when David was required to go to the Middle East for a year in connection with his job. At first the letters came regularly, as David found new and exciting things to share with Jan. However, after the first three months or so, the letters began to come with less regularity. David was having trouble finding new things to write about in his letters and felt as though he was saying the same things over and over again and was being boring.

Jan was wondering why the letters had slowed down. Since she was not in the new location, the Middle East had never had a chance to become ordinary and boring for her. It still seemed as new and as exciting as it had been when she and David had talked about it before he had left. Rather jealously she began to think that David must be having a great time, and maybe even had a lover. She could not understand his reluctance to give details in the few letters she did receive.

She soon found that she would become angry when a long-awaited letter did not contain an answer she wanted even after she had asked for one in two or three consecutive letters. Then when she did get the answer, David would continue to answer the same question over and over again, and would sound more and more angry while seemingly ignoring any new questions she asked.

Stephanie was not helping much either. She had once more begun to suck her thumb; and after Jan had spent many months to get her trained, she found that Stephanie had broken toilet training shortly after David's departure.

The final straw came on a Tuesday afternoon. Jan had just received a letter from David complaining that she was still asking questions which he had already answered and then went on to ask for the fourth time if a certain bill had been paid. On top of that, Stephanie had not stopped crying all morning and now Jan found that the car battery was dead and would have to be replaced. It seemed that they had less money with David away and now she would have to be responsible for yet another thing which David was supposed to be here doing.

When Stephanie's school nurse made a visit to check what was happening following one or two problems reported from school, both Jan and Stephanie were found sitting at the kitchen table crying. After Stephanie had been quieted and they had shared a cup of tea, Jan began to talk about the way she had begun to feel over the past few months. Knowing that at times it is important just to listen and not interrupt, the nurse let Jan continue until she finished. Then they set about looking at the situation as objectively as possible. They set up a realistic timetable for expecting a response to a question based on how long it took one of her letters to get to David and then for one of his to

*get back to her. They made a log of questions which she had asked or
wanted to ask David with columns for the date she asked it, and the
date when he finally responded, so that she wouldn't ask the same
question before he had a chance to answer it. Finally, Jan was helped to
realize that there was nothing 'wrong' with her, and that Stephanie's
loss of toilet training was not unexpected in the circumstances. Jan also
realized that asking for help did not mean that she was in any way less
of a 'good' person.*

*Over the next few weeks Jan talked things over more and more with
the nurse, and slowly became more self-assured and calm. Stephanie
regained her toilet training, and soon Jan and David had re-established
through their letters the good relationship that they had had when he
first left.*

Disruption through divorce

Not all people who are separated will be reunited. For some, complete
separation may be the wisest course of action. Many separations, however, may never be complete, in that there will be common ties that will
continue to keep the couple in contact on a more or less regular basis.
A divorce in which children are involved is the obvious example,
especially when both parents want to keep as full a relationship as
possible with the children. Maintenance requirements and access rights
are not just pieces of paper left behind in the courtroom. Often the
former partners are thrown together, albeit briefly, on a recurring basis.

However, feelings do not always end with courtroom divorce proceedings. The anger and mistrust that may have led to or was generated
by the divorce proceedings can continue for a substantial period of time
or in some cases for ever. The tendency for the parents to use the
children to find out what the other is doing is a subtle way of playing 'one
upmanship'. The child in the centre is cast in a 'no-win' role. No matter
which parent is asking, or what they are asking about, the information is
generally seen by the child as spying. While the parent may be glad to be
rid of that 'chauvinist pig' or that 'constant nag', the child is being forced
to spy on a father or mother. The nurse who walks into the middle of
such a situation may find very entrenched positions.

Acting as an intermediary and staying impartial in domestic situations is
a difficult job. Try never to be cast in a supporting role for either side.
This includes not siding with the parent against the child. As long as
there is no bodily harm imminent, then hearing what a speaker has to say
may be all that is needed to defuse the situation. If the problem is beyond

your ability, then helping to find the appropriate resources such as a lawyer, a marriage guidance counsellor, a doctor or the Citizens' Advice Bureau will be useful.

Children and divorce

Children will inevitably have problems of adjustment with their parents' separation. When we are born, it takes a while to figure out that those two small things out there are feet and that we really do control them. As we grow older, we find many things in our world that we control. Like our parents, for instance. Every time we cry, they will, sooner or later, feed us or clean us or do whatever we want to make us happy. So, as children, we grow up as the centre of our own worlds. Everything centres around us and we control everything to a very considerable extent. So if my parents get a divorce, whose fault is it? Perhaps it is mine. Perhaps if I had not asked for so much, or if I had not been so mean to my brother or sister, or if I had just fed my pet hamster as I had promised when we got it . . . No matter why it happened, you can be sure that a young child will often feel some responsibility for the divorce. It may fall to the nurse to help sort that out.

It is also fairly common to see children playing off one parent against the other. In our culture, children are often rewarded for being good by being given a sweet or something similar. It is no wonder then that when a child is trying to make sure that parents still care it is a material thing that the child seeks, such as toys or gifts. An object or gift is proof that can be held in the hand that the other person still cares. Unfortunately, it is often easier for a person to give things than it is to give love. If a present is equated with love in the eyes of a young child, receiving something becomes very important. After all, the child loves both parents, but if Mum and Dad no longer love each other, what are the chances that they will still love me, especially if I feel that I may, in some ways, be responsible? This helps to explain why children often become very demanding when parents are divorcing or separating. Seeing things from the child's point of view may make it a lot easier to understand why a normally nice child has suddenly become withdrawn or manipulative. This may well be something that you can explain to a distressed parent.

Adults and divorce

Children are not the only ones to experience such feelings. Adults involved in a divorce will often find themselves feeling both guilty and angry, as well as experiencing a decrease in self-esteem. Since we were all children at some time, we have all experienced the idea that the good are rewarded. When we are ending a relationship, even a destructive one, we often feel less than 'good'. Most people feel pretty miserable when they are going through a divorce, and may spend a lot of time alternately blaming themselves and their spouse. Other reactions are many and varied. Some people try to make themselves feel better by going out and 'splurging' on themselves; others may get involved in a new relationship, even if only transitory. Some people will become sexually promiscuous for a time, while others may turn to drink. Yet others struggle alone with feelings of sadness and a sense of failure.

While in some cases children may feel responsible for their parents' divorce, the parents may also be *too* strongly concerned about the children's feelings. Many couples have stayed together in less than the best of situations 'because of the children'. The most serious case is where one spouse (usually the woman) is being subjected to physical or mental abuse. Helping a parent, either husband or wife, to assess whether the termination of a marriage like this might be the best thing for all concerned is difficult, although very necessary. Divorce is especially difficult to contemplate when the split entails a loss of income, or decreased contact with the children, and it is also hard because of the sadness, sense of failure and guilt. However, it is also true that for some people divorce may well be the best option for long-term happiness.

The new problem: Step-parenting

Another very difficult time for most children after a divorce or the death of a parent is when either or both parents start going out with another potential partner. This becomes especially hard for the children as they realize that it is even less likely that their parents will get back together again. It may have been unlikely that they would have got back together anyway, but with someone new in the picture the possibility becomes even more remote.

There is also the problem for the children of their father or mother being 'replaced' by someone new. It is bad enough if one of your parents leaves the family, but then to have a stranger enter brings the whole idea of security within the family into question again. It may appear to the child that if either Mum or Dad can be replaced so easily then their own position must also be somewhat insecure. As the child tries to find a new role in the changing family the presence of a new person requires yet another change.

This can become even worse in the mind of the child as the parent begins spending more and more time with the new adult. Time that used to be given to the child is now reduced by the presence of the new person, and the role that children often assume, because of the separation, as 'Mum's protector' or 'Daddy's little girl' is seen by the child as being taken over by the new adult. Questions such as: 'What do I call this new person?' and 'Must I do what he says?' become very important for the child. Often the child will attempt to do naughty things in order to find out what limits will be set by the new partner. Any disagreement between the two adults may be interpreted by the child as a sign that Mum and Dad may yet get back together, and the child may try unconsciously but apparently deliberately to split up the new partnership.

The adults themselves often have difficulties in this area. 'How will my children react to my new friend?' and 'Will the children like me?' are very common questions asked by many adults as first meetings with children are about to occur. It becomes even more difficult if both of the adults have children of their own. The children in such situations must try to get used to the possibility of step brothers and sisters as well as the possibility of a new parent. There is, in addition, the problem of discipline for the new couple. The question of how to bring up children is not easy for parents who start out together, let alone for those who join the family along the way.

Problems such as these are becoming more and more frequent within our society, and the role of the community nurse is such that no nurse can long remain aloof from them. Attempting to explain the decisions and actions of adults to children sometimes becomes the responsibility of the community nurse and can be even more difficult than helping adults to understand other adults. Your approach will in part be decided by how old the child is, but it can be done reasonably well if two crucial points are borne in mind:

- The most important thing to remember is that children are people, too. As such, they can understand many things if they are given enough time to develop and absorb a realistic explanation. Obviously what is appropriate for a 15-year-old is not necessarily the same for a five-year-old, but that does not mean that the five-year-old should not have some opportunity to explore what is going on.

- But the second thing to note is that this needs to be in a framework where you are not critical of either of the parents to the child. The child will probably feel considerable loyalty to the parents, even if those parents have been hurtful or even cruel. Hence your criticism will be probably prevent any hope of a trusting relationship between you and the child.

When Scott and Stacie's parents got divorced, the children went to live with their mother. Everything went well until Mrs Brown brought home a 'special friend'. As their mother's relationship with her new friend got stronger and stronger, Scott began to leave home earlier each night and stay out later. He brought his friends home less often and when he did, they stayed for shorter and shorter periods of time. At the same time, Stacie began to spend more time in her room alone. Mrs Brown was not particularly concerned by their behaviour. In fact, she was pleased to have the time to get to know her new friend and to spend more time with him. By the time she realized that the children were behaving differently, she could not understand what it was that had brought about the change.

For a few weeks she tried ringing up the children's father and getting him to come over and discipline them, but each time he tried it seemed to have almost the opposite effect from what was wanted. Scott seemed to get more uncontrollable and Stacie withdrew more into her room. Finally, their mother consulted their family doctor, and a health visitor visited the home.

After getting to know the children and gaining their confidence, the nurse was able to help explain to the children what was happening. She pointed out that they were still a very real part of their mother's life, and also helped them to accept that while their mother's friend was special to her, their own father was not being 'replaced' and would still be their father. At the same time, the health visitor was able to explain to Mrs Brown what the children were experiencing and what their fears were. This enabled Mrs Brown to discuss the situation with both the children's father and her new boyfriend, and to find ways for all of them to reassure the children that they were still loved and wanted. This proved to be a very effective intervention on the part of the nurse in a rather tricky situation.

Disruption through abandonment: "Frankly my dear. . . ."

Clark Gable's reply became a catch phrase when he stood at the bottom of the stairs and told Scarlet O'Hara that he was leaving her. Such things just did not happen to 'good' people. The only time someone left a family was when there was a specific reason, and one partner or other could always be held responsible. So if someone does leave, not only is the family a failure (and by association everyone within it), but someone must be to blame.

While that might be true in the cinema, it is not often true in real life. Although the idea persists, and questions such as 'Was it my fault?' and 'What did I do?' will often be asked by whoever is left behind, sometimes people do just leave: the one who is left is not necessarily at fault. The person who has left may have individual and very personal reasons for leaving, or it may be that this particular relationship simply did not work. Even if the one leaving does blame the person left behind, say perhaps in a note, what was written is not necessarily true.

If the person leaving gives no reason, then the imagination of those left behind can run wild. In such cases, it may be very difficult for a third party, such as a nurse, to ease the burden of guilt for those left.

Christopher, a district nurse, was seeing a family to care for the grandmother when Kevin, one of the teenage children, left home leaving a note behind that just said, 'I'm leaving'. The family's worry about whether he was all right was bad enough, but added to this was their self-blame. In fact, this became the major problem. Kevin's mother blamed herself and wouldn't stop talking about it. Every time Christopher called to see the grandmother, it was the first thing Kevin's mother would talk about. Kevin's father, on the other hand, refused to even mention it. It was almost as though it was illegal to discuss the teenager, and each time his wife or Christopher tried to talk to him about it, he would stop the conversation immediately. While Christopher was never able to get the father to discuss the matter, his visits and subsequent talks with the mother went a long way towards helping the family cope with the fact that one of the children had left home in that manner. Christopher could then spend more time looking after the grandmother again.

Disruption through death

Leaving home is not the only way in which a member might be removed from the family. Death is an irreversible leaving, though it results in more complications if that death is self-chosen by suicide. Because death is such an important topic, we have already devoted an entire chapter to it, so will not go into detail again here except to observe that while most deaths happen to the elderly, situations such as the death of a child or a stillbirth can be especially devastating. With the changes in family structure that result there will be a change in relationships. Family members may become closer or move farther apart, but a change of some sort will inevitably occur.

Both death and intentional leaving are combined in suicide. The tendency for recrimination by the family members, along with the finality of the death, makes suicide one of the most extreme traumas a family can face. While it may seem that suicide would have been more appropriately discussed in the chapter on death, it forms the ultimate case of a disrupted family since it is a choice made by the individual rather than something that just happens. We therefore discuss it here.

Most people consider life to be precious and to be preserved at all costs. Strong religious, medical and social pressures continually re-inforce this view in Western culture, and in consequence the decision to take one's own life is difficult for many people to comprehend. In the minds of many people it is assumed that just as there must be someone to blame for a divorce, so also there surely must be somebody to blame for a suicide; since no one 'in their right mind' would commit suicide, it must be the fault of those left behind.

Common sense does not always form the basis of the decisions and ideas held by people who are suffering. Many of the feelings which any bereaved person has will be present, but added to these will be both guilt and anger. Following a suicide, it is particularly important to let the bereaved express their anger at what the person committing suicide has done to them, and not to let 'respect for the dead' or guilt stand in the way of this very important emotion. As always, a fine line has to be trodden between allowing the people left behind to talk out feelings and fears, and encouraging someone to wallow in self-pity, despair and bitterness.

While this can generally be accomplished by maintaining a sense of reality about the patient and the circumstances surrounding the suicide, the nurse's personal ideas and religious or moral judgements must not be forced upon anyone. If the nurse feels that the situation is more than can be handled easily, other, more appropriate agencies can be found. Knowing your limits as a nurse can be one of the most helpful assets for any family you are working with. It is the ability to distinguish between where you can and cannot help that marks a sensitive nurse from those who, even with the best intentions, 'rush in where angels fear to tread'.

CONCLUDING COMMENTS

The family is not always a haven of love and security. Nor does every family fit the traditional breakfast cereal packet image of smiling father, mother and two happy, contented and secure children. For some the family is a battleground, whilst for others it merely represents a sense of failure and guilt. Each family is unique. Do not let your own ideas of what is best dominate either your assessment or your intervention, but be prepared to offer support and encouragement to people who are often struggling on the front line with the changes that are going on throughout our society.

Suggestions for further reading

Skynner, R. and Cleese, J. (1983) *Families and How to Survive Them*. London: Methuen.
  Written by the well-known comedian John Cleese and Robin Skynner the family therapist. It is an entertaining and readable book on family life, which also has a serious message about how to help families in trouble. Good cartoons.

Tizard, B. (1977) *Adoption: A second chance*. London: Open Books.
  The story of a group of adopted children and the consequences and problems associated with adoption. It is both well written and optimistic, and would be helpful to anyone working with adoption or who has some personal interest in it.

Wallerstein, J.S. and Kelly, J.B. (1980) *Surviving the Breakup: How children and parents cope with divorce*. London: Grant McIntyre.
  A detailed discussion of many of the difficult questions surrounding divorce like what to tell the children, whether they will be permanently harmed by the experience, and how contact with the absent parent should be maintained. Useful for both parents and nurses.

Walrond-Skinner, S. (1979) *Family and Marital Psychotherapy*. London: Routledge and Kegan Paul.
  Although fairly advanced and technical in its approach, this book is well worth a look if you want to know more about how families function, and why they sometimes go wrong. Treatment approaches are also discussed.

Chapter 7

Sex and the Patient

The most private of all interactions, sex may be the most confusing as well as the most pleasurable. It can also be the most secretive, bounded by ignorance and fear. Thus it is very hard to know what is 'normal' or what is 'acceptable'. Nurses are often seen as experts on the subject, by virtue of their priveleged professional access to the human body. In fact, most nurses know no more about sex than what comes from their personal experience, for people confuse knowing about reproduction with knowing about sex.

In this chapter we look at some of the issues and concerns that nurses may encounter in day-to-day interactions with patients when the topic of sex crops up:

1. Situations when nurses may feel discomfort at being the 'unbiased and neutral expert' on a subject where they may actually feel a little unsure or have strong personal feelings.

2. The situation where the nurse has to be extremely sensitive to the patients' feelings of vulnerability and fear, and therefore may need special skills despite having had very little training.

Both of these sorts of difficulty tend to crop up in all of the areas which we consider in this chapter – sex education, pregnancy and abortion, sexual problems, the menopause and sexually transmitted diseases.

TALKING ABOUT SEX

Talking about sex is not something that most people find easy, especially if what they need is sex education. People (including many nurses) often assert that if sex is so common and basic to humanity then obviously

83

everyone knows what to do and how do it. If I do not, then there must be something 'wrong' with me. Therefore, I will be very cautious about letting anyone know how 'strange' or deficient I am. By the time I am in enough discomfort to broach the subject, I am likely to be extremely sensitive to any possibility that the nurse might be laughing at me or may be shocked by what I say.

This problem becomes even more acute when the nurse and the patient are of opposite sexes. Not only is there the difficulty of admitting a lack of knowledge or understanding, but the nurse may be seen as a potential, although relatively unlikely, sexual partner. To talk about something as sensitive as sex to someone who may (at some future date) be able to respond to it is very threatening. If people fear that they may be 'deficient', the last thing they will want is to have that fear confirmed by someone who could be able to judge.

It is this fear which nurses need to be aware of when answering questions. The best thing is to try to answer questions accurately without confirming the idea that there is something 'wrong' or deficient about the patient. Equally essential is the ability to let the patient know that the subject is acceptable, and not 'dirty' or 'sinful'.

Common sense is enough in most cases to remind the nurse of the importance of the surroundings for such discussions. There needs to be privacy when talking about sex. For example, if you are visiting a family where a disabled young person needs bathing, you may become aware that the young person has something that he or she wants to talk about. First establish whether any parent is to be invited into the discussion. In some cases to exclude a parent would be to miss a chance to create the opportunity of later discussion between parent and adolescent. In other circumstances the young person might feel that privacy has been destroyed if he or she was not ready to discuss a difficult matter with a parent. Often neither parent nor adolescent will have words with which they feel comfortable, so that the first task may be to talk about the words that are to be used.

Try not to deluge the patient with a flood of information, though. To go from having insufficient knowledge to having too much is jumping from the frying pan into the fire: the result is still confusion. That fine line between too little and too much knowledge is one that must be worked out by the nurse and patient in each situation. There is no need to get everything said in one go. Follow-up discussions can be used to check on what the patient has understood and the effectiveness of any suggestions that the nurse may have made.

BUT DON'T WE ALL KNOW EVERYTHING THERE IS TO KNOW ABOUT SEX?

The answer to this question is no. There are lots of groups of people who are very ignorant about the facts of reproduction and sexuality, even in this so-called 'permissive' society. For example, mothers sometimes fail to inform their daughters about what to expect from the onset of puberty, so that when the girl first finds blood on her underwear, it is a big shock. In Coleen McCulloch's *The Thorn Birds*, Meggie's discovery of her first period leads her to think, in terror, that she is suffering from some terrible disease and is very likely to die. She suffers in silence and confusion for several days, until she is told about the facts of menstruation by the priest. Such an experience is still not infrequent.

Ideas about the 'dirtiness' or 'danger' of monthly bleeding can still crop up. Some mothers may tell their daughters that they should not swim, dance, play sport or even wash their hair while having their periods. Some cultures, for example orthodox Muslims and some orthodox Jews, believe that a woman should not prepare food while menstruating. Respecting the cultural and religious beliefs of your patients whilst wanting to make clear what Western medical science understands about such matters may be very difficult. Girls can be gently informed that they can do whatever they feel like doing during their periods, so long as they are happy and do not feel uncomfortable. If religious observance forbids particular acts there is no reason why the observance should be related to inaccurate facts.

The discovery of the ways in which sex takes place can be quite frightening, if someone does not know what to expect. Again, in *The Thorn Birds*, Meggie's first experience of sex is so unexpected and so strange that she feels nothing but fear and horror at what her new husband is doing to her. It is not true that 'everyone knows the facts of life'. Where do all the parts go? What are you supposed to do? These may seem naïve questions, but to someone who has never had the opportunity to look closely at the sexual parts of the opposite sex they are very real ones.

One fairly common complaint presented to family planning clinics is failure to consummate the marriage. And it is not just newly-wed couples who have this difficulty. A couple may come for help after years of misery, simply because they desperately want to conceive a child, and so discover information that their confusion and uncertainty have previously denied them. It is by no means unknown that infertility clinics may appear to take an adequate sexual history on the basis that 'everyone knows', but then engage in extensive testing when in fact insertion is not actually taking place. This can happen because the questioning to establish whether or not intercourse is taking place has not been specific enough. Terms like 'making love' are too vague as the basis for establishing clinical facts, and words that come from Latin, like 'intercourse', are often not properly understood by patients. On the other hand, nurses and doctors may not know the words the patient knows.

There may of course be other reasons for the non-consummation of marriage. One or both partners may feel so much fear or disgust at the very idea of sex that insertion is completely out of the question. Also, one or both partners may have some particular difficulty with becoming (or staying) aroused which makes love-making almost impossible. Later in this chapter, we look at specific sexual difficulties, and also suggest some ways of helping which nurses can use.

The idea is also still around that masturbation is wrong and will cause physical or mental harm to anyone who practices it. It is not very long since children's hands were tied up when going to bed to stop them from touching themselves sexually, and some children were even subjected to mutilating surgery to stop the practice. Parents need to be informed by the health professionals that there is no evidence whatever that masturbation is harmful. On the contrary: it is one very satisfactory way in which sexual needs can be satisfied. Parents are often worried if their children do seem to be extremely interested in their sexual parts, and play 'doctors and nurses' with other children. In the vast majority of cases, this is simply natural curiosity, and the parents should simply be reassured that there will be no lasting harm unless they themselves create it by making such curiosity appear less natural than it is. Children do, however, need some guidance here. Not all children want to play these games, and the first crucial lesson about the right to say 'no' to unwanted invasiveness can be taught. A person's body is their own, and the child has to realize that he or she can refuse to join in. In addition, children need to be taught that there is a time and place for such activities, and that intimate physical behaviour is not really acceptable in public.

FEELINGS ABOUT SEX

When talking about sex, encourage an approach to sex which supports the belief that it is a normal, enjoyable and healthy part of being human. Because people are so sensitive about this topic patients are often quick to pick up any hint on the nurse's part that, as they had feared, sex is dirty, or worse, that they are ridiculous for being ignorant about it. That means that you, as a nurse, must spend at least some time thinking profession-ally about sex, so that you do not give these messages to patients. How were you told about the 'facts of life'? Did your mother or father suggest to you that sex was something bad or dangerous? Did your parents and teachers punish you for being curious? We know from research that parents often convey their hidden anxieties to their children. Nurses can do the same to their patients.

When the nurse is requested to give information to someone else (for example, when an embarrassed parent hands over the task of giving sex education to a mentally handicapped young person, or to a curious but apparently ignorant son or daughter), knowing what the other person knows or feels becomes even more essential. The problem here is two-fold. The child or young person often possesses information, much of which may well be inaccurate. This needs to be sorted out and accurate information offered. The second problem is that if parents do not give their children much information about sex they probably do not give them clear guidance on responsibility issues either. So then you may have to offer guidance as if you were a parent, which may leave you feeling quite a long way out of your depth.

DIFFICULT DECISIONS: PREGNANCY AND ABORTION

Much has been said already about the need for the nurse to be sensitive to the patient's feelings and reactions. But this can only come from self-awareness regarding your own feelings and values. As outsiders and experts, nurses often have a perspective that the patient will not have. While it is important for nurses to be able to share those ideas and perceptions with the patient, they also have to be careful not to push the patient towards any particular course of action. Nowhere is this more true than with the topics of contraception, pregnancy and abor-tion.

Subjects may have to be discussed which challenge the beliefs of either the nurse or the patient. For example, nurses may be asked to give advice on whether or not homosexuality should be permitted. They may also be asked about the morality of contraception or abortion. As far as possible, the nurse should decline to give personal opinions on these topics, not only because it really is not up to the nurse to make decisions about patients' lives, but also because it may give the patient a source of blame for anything he or she may later have second thoughts about. The ability to present alternatives whilst leaving the final decision to the patient is essential.

There are times, of course, as every nurse knows, when some painful decisions *have* to be made. In these cases, the nurse should probably aim to support the patient as far as possible in whatever the patient decides. An example of this type of situation is the young woman who finds herself pregnant against her wishes. Parental approval and support may have been withheld, or, more frequently, may not even have been sought, since the young woman may have been afraid to approach her parents. For some, termination of pregnancy may be the best alternative, although few patients choose this option lightly. The available evidence suggests that women who have abortions do not usually suffer from any long-term consequences, either physically or emotionally, although at the time the decision can be extremely painful. But in the weeks following the termination, feelings of loss, guilt and rage may persist. Support at this stage is immensely valuable.

For those who make the decision to keep the baby, there may be an even greater need for support. The first thing to do is to try and help the young woman to understand her present feelings. If she sees herself as being punished for having done something wrong, she may feel unable to accept the support of friends or relatives. Likewise, if she sees the pregnancy as a case of having been 'caught', she may well attempt to conceal or hide it from friends or relatives for as long as possible. It is not too difficult to recall a time when young girls who were found to be pregnant were sent away so that the neighbours would not find out. That idea still persists in some parts of society, so that the opinions of the neighbours and hiding the guilt of the family seem to be more important than the health and happiness of the new mother and baby.

Your role as the nurse in this situation must be to offer professional support and encouragement, as you would to any pregnant woman. But it is important to realize that a woman with an unplanned pregnancy may have all sorts of complicated feelings of guilt, regret, anger and apprehension which are less likely in the married woman. You may become a central figure in her life for a while, although you should clearly encourage her to seek the help of her family and social network as much as possible.

Pregnancy problems do not only happen to the young and single, however. There is a growing group of women who have decided either that they do not want children or that they have had as many as they want. Sometimes these women may also find themselves alone and without support if their husbands and/or families *do* want another child. They too will need a lot of support from the nursing services. If, under pressure, a woman agrees to a pregnancy about which she is ambivalent, not only will it affect her but it will also affect the entire family socially, economically and emotionally. Child care facilities may have to be found or extended; money set aside for holidays, home improvements or just paying off debts will have to be redirected; and, just when freedom was within sight, a child arrives who will demand the total support of the mother again. It is understandable that even after apparent agreement, a great deal of anger may also be present. This will be even more true if the pregnancy was the result of failed contraception.

With the exception of abstinence, the highly unreliable rhythm method and the sheath, most forms of birth control tend to have some connection with the health service. Contraception is usually prescribed, fitted, dispensed or otherwise suggested and endorsed by someone who is seen to be a part of the health service. As a representative of that service (even if you had nothing to do with actually recommending the contraception) much of the uncertainty or anger which a patient feels in regard to an unplanned pregnancy due to failed contraception may be directed towards you. Recognizing and dealing with that anger may be necessary before any useful relationship with the patient can be achieved. As we have said already, the best way for the nurse to deal with anger such as this is to listen to what the patient is saying, try not to become defensive in response, and then to help the patient to talk herself into constructively recognizing the undeniable fact of her pregnancy. It is only at this point that the patient will be able to make a sensible decision about what to do.

There are also cases in which a woman may happily find herself pregnant but also have very mixed feelings about the expected child, as where there is a fear of hereditary problems or some genetic anomaly. Sometimes just knowing that tests are available to determine whether or not a problem exists is sufficient to reduce the anxiety. It is important to make use of the period between the discovery of the pregnancy and the date of the test to establish a solid working relationship with the patient. As the date of the test draws near, the nurse can expect that any anxiety that does exist will rise to new heights. It is during this period of uncertainty that the nurse can, and often does, become a primary source of support for the pregnant woman. This usually happens because the nurse is seen in the role of expert, as well as, in most cases, being a woman herself.

When positive test results are received the issue of terminating the pregnancy arises again. As we have already said, abortion is not only distressing for most women but can also give rise to strong emotions in the nurse. This is especially likely if the nurse has strong religious or moral views regarding termination, or if the nurse has undergone similar decisions in the past and has not been happy with what happened.

Trying to maintain a sense of neutrality is not easy in the best of situations. Attempting to do so with a topic as emotionally laden as abortion is as difficult as it is important. Although it sounds like a contradiction, often the best way to remain neutral is to be very aware of your own feelings on the subject. If the nurse is involved in a discussion on whether or not to recommend an abortion and does not admit these feelings at least to him or herself, then that nurse may not be able to give unbiased advice. For example, if the nurse states a neutral position and in the process of the discussion it becomes apparent that his or her position is not neutral, then the credibility of the nurse has been destroyed or, at best, severely strained.

If you feel really unable to keep your opinions to yourself, then the best thing may be to say what you feel, but make it clear that your intention is not to influence the patient's decision. This is not to say that the nurse has to tell everyone every opinion at all times, but if the patient is to rely on the nurse for counsel and support, there must also be trust and honesty as an important part of that relationship. Finding ways of conveying the complexity of your own feelings, even as an expert, will bring nothing but benefit to a patient, so long as you make it equally clear that you are not expecting the other person to accept your opinion as the 'right' opinion simply because of who you are.

This does not mean that once an opinion has been voiced all neutrality is lost. A professional training carries an obligation to let the patient know as much as possible about the decision that has to be made. For example, the nurse who is morally opposed to abortion should not mislead the pregnant mother by scare stories about possible effects of the abortion: it is now known that most women are not damaged psychologically or physically by termination of pregnancy if they are offered plenty of support. But nor should the nurse who very actively supports a 'woman's right to choose' minimize the traumatic effects that having an abortion can have on, say, a very religious person. The important point to remember is not which way the patient decides or whether the patient alone has the right to make that decision, but that as far as possible the patient feels that the best decision has been made, and is supported by the medical and nursing staff around her.

Although we have talked exclusively about the mother in this section, the father will also have complex feelings about the pregnancy, and this is not to be forgotten in the discussions and decisions that take place. Make sure you always ask the father to join you if at all possible, and if he cannot or will not, endeavour to find out the reasons. These could have a significant bearing on the kind of help the mother-to-be needs.

BUT WHAT ABOUT SEXUAL DIFFICULTIES?

Surveys have shown that most people at some point in their lives have some sort of difficulty in their sexual relationships. These problems spread throughout the age range, and occur as both fairly short-term difficulties (a lack of desire on the part of the woman after childbirth, for example), and as fairly long-term problems (the prolonged inability on the part of the man to maintain an erection for any length of time, for example). These difficulties are not only very worrying because they threaten very important things, but, as sex is a central part of life for most of us, when it goes wrong it often creates the sense that there is something very wrong about us.

Both partners in a relationship are affected by a sexual difficulty even if it seems that only one has the 'problem'. The kind of questions that run through people's minds are:

- 'Does this mean I am not a proper man any more?'
- 'Am I a failure in my marriage?'
- 'Doesn't my husband find me attractive any more?'
- 'Is she having an affair with someone else?'

Such questions, upsetting as they are, may not always be put into words by patients, nor have been said by the partners to each other, except perhaps as angry accusations. The nurse has to know that such fears and feelings are quite possibly there, hidden beneath the surface, even if the patient has difficulty talking about them.

So what can a nurse do? Although a number of specialized clinics and services do exist where the staff are trained to provide sexual and marital therapy through the health service, the community nurse is well placed to provide the simplest, and often the most effective form of treatment for sexual difficulties: reassurance, knowledge and support.

The first thing that must be done, however, is to ensure that there is no biological or physiological cause for the problem. Sexual problems may be the first indication of potentially serious conditions such as diabetes, or they may be a side-effect of current medication, as in some of the drugs commonly given for high blood pressure or the management of anxiety. Once it is known that no physical cause exists, however, often just knowing that such problems are very widespread can help. The picture presented in films and on television of the sexually active man, who is always interested in sex, and who is always successful in giving ecstatic sexual experiences to a succession of women (often by carrying out a physical routine which would not shame an Olympic athlete) is, of course, far from the truth. But to admit that *you* do not behave like that in bed may be very difficult. Hence men (and it is usually men, because women seem to be better at sharing their feelings of 'inadequacy' with one another) may not realize that it is quite normal not to want sex all the time, and that erections do not just happen 'on demand'. For women, if you are tired or worried about something else, then it is not surprising you do not feel interested in sex. Just knowing that can sometimes help.

Another important piece of information which can be of enormous assistance to people with worries about sex is the role played by anxiety in making things worse. It simply is not possible for either a man or a woman to get sexually aroused if they are 'watching' themselves to see if they will get an erection, have an orgasm or be 'good enough'.

Elizabeth, who had requested help for her ageing father, had been having routine visits from her community nurse. One day, as the nurse was preparing to leave, Elizabeth asked the nurse if she could ask a very private question. Nervously, she said that for the last six months she and her husband Ben had not had sex. When the nurse asked Elizabeth how this had all started Elizabeth said that one night Ben had come home from the pub, after celebrating a friend's promotion, and had started to make love to Elizabeth. However, he very soon lost his erection, and, mortified, rolled over and pretended to be asleep. The following night he again tried, after visiting the pub for some Dutch courage. By the time he and Elizabeth went to bed Ben was so anxious about his forthcoming performance that again nothing happened. Feeling humiliated twice in a row, Ben refused to attempt again rather than risk failing a third time. In order not to feel that there was something inherently wrong with himself, he told Elizabeth that she was to blame for not being 'exciting' enough. Since this was not actually the basic problem, she was in a 'no win' position. No matter what she did, Ben's anxiety over another possible 'failure' prevented him from responding in a natural, relaxed manner and thereby obtaining a satisfactory erection. This, in turn, reinforced her worry that it might, after all, be her fault.

After meeting them and verifying that there was no medical problem, the nurse was able to explain that Ben's initial difficulty was a common reaction to large quantities of alcohol. She further explained how his anxiety had interfered with subsequent attempts. By discussing the subject openly and freely, Ben came to realize that not all men matched the image that he had been led to believe in. By helping Ben and Elizabeth focus on what was happening rather than what they thought should be happening, the nurse allowed them to put aside any concerns

about 'performance' or desirability and enjoy themselves as they were.
Gradually, the anxiety vanished and was replaced by a healthy and
mutually satisfying relationship, which was actually more pleasurable to
them than it had been before the 'problem' had occurred.

Not all sexual difficulties are so recent in origin or straightforward and some must be referred to appropriate therapists. Nevertheless, the community nurse is in a good position to prevent many problems from getting to the point where more formal referral is required.

SEX AND THE DISABLED

Community nurses can be of particular help in the sexual problems of the disabled. Physical disabilities (arising, for example, from severe arthritis or multiple sclerosis) do not mean that people do not have sexual feelings and needs. In a survey carried out in 1975, it was found that nearly two-thirds of disabled people said they had a problem with sex. Sadly, more people who become disabled (through accidents or illness) get divorced than the average. Also, fewer disabled people than able-bodied people get married in the first place.

Thus a major problem for the physically handicapped is sexual isolation and frustration. In the past it used to be thought that it was not healthy for people who were handicapped to have sexual feelings, so that if a disabled person felt sexually frustrated he or she must be perverted and dirty. Because bodies may be disfigured and not obviously sexually attractive, it is somehow assumed that normal sexual yearnings will be distorted too. This idea still exists in some institutions for the disabled, where no opportunity is provided for people to express their sexual feelings or affirm their sexuality. But it can also exist for the disabled at home where, for example, an unsympathetic or embarrassed family have no realization that a very disabled son might still experience sexual tension and be much happier for some help in experiencing his feelings through masturbation.

It is of particular value in this situation for the nurse to 'give permission' by affirming that masturbation is a healthy and enjoyable act, and to help the family accept that it satisfies a normal human need. It may also be that the community nurse can play a crucial role in suggesting ways for the young person to relieve tensions, for example by using particular positions or mechanical aids. Some nurses may find this difficult or embarrassing through lack of familiarity with how a member of the opposite sex does in fact masturbate. The boundaries of personal and professional knowledge in this area are very blurred. An organization called *Sexual Problems of the Disabled* (286, Camden Road, London N7 OBJ) provides very helpful literature with suggestions of imaginative ways for dealing with situations like this one. Such resources can be used by the community nursing service to broaden the horizon of possibilities.

Most disabled people who do have difficulties say that these difficulties result directly from their physical handicap, such as stiffness of joints, generalized weakness, tremor or spasm during love-making or constant pain. A high proportion of requests for help from the disabled are about sexual positions to use when making love, or for suggestions of alternatives to sexual intercourse.

One of the most sensitive treatments of the subject can be found in the film *Coming Home* where Jon Voight, as a severely disabled Vietnam war veteran, develops a sexual relationship with the character played by Jane Fonda. Their use of alternatives to 'normal' sex in both type and style made millions aware for the first time that relying on a wheelchair for mobility does not mean the end of all sexual desires or contacts. It is an awareness that is, unfortunately, all too easy for many to lose.

A nurse can also encourage partners to talk to each other about the problem. A colostomy operation made necessary because of the discovery of malignant tissues left Steve with a bag which had to be worn at all times, including, of course, in bed. Prior to the operation, Steve and Amy's marriage had been happy enough, although both of them had been a little shy of talking about sex and avoided using any words about their sexual organs except in the most vague and discreet way. When Steve had his operation they stopped having sex. Steve was terrified of the bag bursting during sex, but was unable to confide in Amy because of embarrassment. Amy didn't like to bring up the topic, also because of embarrassment. Only a sensitive question, asked during a routine visit from a nurse, opened up the topic. The nurse, realizing that the main problem seemed to be the lack of communication between the two, talked through the problem with them. By using simple, non-medical language about the sexual organs, she was able to encourage the pair to share their fears with each other, and so to resolve the problem.

SEX AND LATER MATURITY

Just as there is no requirement for people to become sexually active on the day they enter puberty, so likewise there is no reason for them to cease being sexual upon the arrival of menopause. Unfortunately some men and women still see the menopause as a termination of their sexual life together, and so the idea that reproduction and sexuality are not irretrievably linked still comes as a surprise to many. As hormone levels alter and her body changes, a woman may feel out of control or uncertain why she acts and feels the way she does. Any increase in sexual drive may be seen by the woman as being wrong or abnormal. Discovering that this is actually quite normal may be extremely important for her. Here the nurse has an important task in reassuring the patient that sexuality is an essential part of life, which can continue to bring her pleasure and intimacy right to the end of life.

It may also help a wife and a husband to discover the difference between thinking of the menopause as a life change and thinking of it as lifestyle change. The major difference is that while the biological consequences of the menopause are largely out of the patient's control, the lifestyle changes it offers can give the patient an increase in control over her life and what she does with it. In other words, her physical changes do not mean that she is no longer a 'complete' woman; merely that she is now free from having to worry about possible pregnancy in the future. Here the nurse's own feelings about sex may also be important. Ask yourself if you feel that it is all right for older people to enjoy sex. If you feel that it is not, ask yourself where this idea comes from, whether it is a rational feeling. Doubts about older people enjoying sexual intimacy may be linked to what you feel about your own parents having sex.

In talking about the menopause, questions of 'the male menopause' often crop up. While no actual equivalent to the female menopause has ever been proved in men, the nurse will be told of instances of decreased sexual desire or ability in men. The reasons for this may be physical or psychological, or a mixture of the two. In every case it is important to encourage the patient to have the cause investigated by a doctor who is an expert in sexual medicine. It is also important to remember that, as with the menopause in women, a problem in bed can both cause and be caused by feelings of depression. Retirement or unemployment may occur at the same time as the man's awareness of his decreasing ability to get and keep an erection, and these events can be cumulative in threatening his sense of himself as a man. He may not be able to put these feelings into words, but if you notice, while visiting a family where the husband is unemployed, that the wife is making digs at her husband's 'manhood', you might explore the possibility that he could be feeling inadequate in bed as well as in the world of work.

THE WORM IN THE APPLE . . .

A final word needs to be said on the subject of sexually transmitted diseases. While it is OK to have a cold, the measles or even cancer, in our society it is not 'acceptable' to contract a venereal disease. In other words, VD is highly stigmatized. Because of this, people are often very ignorant about it, and do not know how to recognize symptoms. This obviously slows down or prevents the discovery of the disease. More unfortunately, it can also stop someone who knows he or she has a venereal disease from doing something about it.

In an area where there is probably even more a sense of being caught or punished than in unwanted pregnancies, it becomes increasingly important for the nurse to be accepting and non-judgemental while strongly encouraging the patient to seek medical help. Not only is this important for the patient's own health, but it could also affect the health of partners or future children. People can often be persuaded to do things because they feel others would approve of them for doing it, even if they will not do it for themselves.

Sally, a new mother who was being seen for a series of injections by a community nurse, refused to go to the special clinic with what appeared to the nurse to be symptoms of a sexually transmitted disease. Sally said she wouldn't go because she was frightened of being spotted there by friends. The nurse asked Sally to think what her new baby son Michael would think of her for not safeguarding her own health. While Michael was obviously not old enough at the time to consider the question, by adding to the discussion an assumption of what his views might have been, the scale was tipped and Sally was persuaded. She went along to the clinic the next day.

CONCLUDING REMARKS

In this chapter we have looked at some of the problems that community nurses are likely to come across as part of their daily routines in dealing with the subject of sex. While it is a subject which is likely to affect everyone, it remains one of the most private, and every effort must be made to maintain the patient's sense of dignity. But at the same time, the nurse often has to encourage the patient to gather new information or explore various alternatives. Comfort about expressing attitudes and ease in using words that are found socially embarrassing will be especially effective in communicating about sexual matters.

Suggestions for further reading

Brown, P.T. and Faulder, C. (1979) *Treat Yourself to Sex: A guide to good loving.* Harmondsworth: Penguin.
> For couples who want to get more out of their sexual relationship, this book is a practical guide to sex and sexual problems. It is both clear and reasonably priced, so worth recommending to patients.

Glover, J. (1985) *Human Sexuality and Nursing Care.* London: Croom Helm.
> Ideal for any nurse who would like clear factual information about sex, sexual problems and sex therapy. It also deals with such subjects as the sexual needs of the handicapped and sexual offences.

Chapter 8

Parenting Problems

Formal education is an essential requirement in most advanced societies. Millions are spent each year to teach young people how to read and write, to do maths and to gain a basic understanding of history and science. After statutory school leaving examinations may come technical training or further study and then for some, it is off to college, polytechnic or university for even more education or professional training. Strangely enough, with all our cultural emphasis on training before starting an occupation, parenting is still seen as something that just comes naturally. Seldom is a young woman instructed in the daily skills needed to become a good mother, and, likewise, men do not seek qualifications in fathering. Of course, we all have our own opinions on what a good parent should be like, and many of these ideas are based on what our own parents did. Some of our ideas may come from our religion and others from general reading or observing others. These are all perfectly valid sources of information and have withstood the test of time. Looking around at the vast majority of parents, it is obvious that the system has worked quite well, since the majority of people appear to do quite adequately as parents.

At the same time there are notable exceptions. Over the past few years the subject of child abuse or baby battering has become more and more common in the daily newspapers. Whether there is more child abuse now than in the past or whether it is just being more openly discussed nowadays is an argument beyond the scope of this book; but that it exists is very evident. It is so important, in fact, that Chapter 9 deals with the subject in detail. This chapter provides some general ideas to alert you to the sort of problems (not involving child abuse) that do crop up in parenting, and where there could be serious consequences for the well-being of either child or parent.

WHERE IT STARTS

It would be very easy to say that difficulties with parenting are the fault
of the previous set of parents, and that if people do not become good
parents it is because they were badly brought by the preceding generation, who in turn were badly brought up by *their* parents, who in turn . . .
But this type of reasoning can be used to blame parents for many
generations back into the past, and still will not help today's young
people learn what to do now. There is a great difference between
playing 'Mummies and Daddies' and actually being a parent. The dolls
that we played with in childhood could be put away when other things
caught our attention or we wanted to be somewhere else doing other
things. You cannot put away a baby when you get bored with it, or when
it will not stop crying.

As we have already said in Chapter 6, it was far more common in the
past to see two, three or even more generations living together in the
same house. This provided a new parent with the opportunity to have a
'resident expert' at hand to help with any crisis that occurred. Because of
the mobility of today's society, extended families tend not to live in the
same house or even in the same town. Parents with young children are
often at the start of their careers and seldom have large incomes. Many
more may not be able to afford babysitters due to the additional burden of
unemployment. Add to this a baby who continues to cry for no apparent
reason, and it is no wonder that almost any parent at some time has
wondered if they are really any good at parenting and whether it is all
worthwhile. Most parenting problems arise from one of three sources.

1. Practical difficulties.
The first is the inability to get the things needed for the child because of
external problems such as a lack of money, or other practical difficulties.
An example could be malnourishment due to the lack of money to buy
appropriate food for an infant. Once a source for either the money or
the food is found the parent can then act effectively. The obvious and
practical can sometimes be neglected by trying to become *too* psychological.

2. Lack of knowledge.
The second form of parenting problem is caused by a lack of knowledge
or skill on the part of the parents. Such parents may well need some
instruction about where to find an item or service, or they may need to
be taught basic parenting skills such as the care and feeding of the infant,
how to tell when the baby is ill, and what they can realistically expect

from their child. It is an error to assume that people automatically know these things just because they were able to conceive a child.

3. Self-confidence.

The third type of problem has to do with the parents' self-confidence and motivation. Some parents may in fact be very frightened by their new babies, and feel petrified by the responsibility of having such a dependent creature all of their own. They may believe that in order to be a parent you have to do every thing right, whatever that implies. Alternatively, other parents may not in fact be very interested in their children, and may not be prepared to try and learn from the experience.

THE MYTHS OF PARENTHOOD

No matter who they are, most parents, sooner or later, have to confront some of the myths of parenthood which often make the job of being a parent much more difficult than need be. Myths such as these can cause considerable misery to both children and parents, and as a nurse working in the community, you may be in a good position to dispel some of them.

The 'It's Natural' myth

The most obvious myth is that parenting comes naturally. It does not. It takes a great deal of effort. By the second or third child, many people have a pretty good idea of what they need to do as parents, but that first child is for many an exercise in trial-and-error learning. We often look at how others perform the job and then compare ourselves with them. When we see all of those other little ones on their best behaviour and *we* are faced with the prime contender for the world record holder of the loudest cry, it is sometimes hard not to doubt our own abilities. After all, we all know how much fun parenting 'should' be. As a consequence our self-confidence as parents takes a considerable knock.

The 'Mothering Instinct' myth

Because mothers historically have spent more time with newborn infants than fathers, it is often assumed that mothers have 'special' knowledge or instincts for child care. But human beings are not like animals, and one of the most important differences is that, unlike animal behaviour, lots of human behaviour is *learned* rather than instinctive. The idea that there is such a thing as a 'mothering instinct' is simply not true. However, because in most cases mothers spend more time with the infant they do generally get to know the new baby better and can, for example, distinguish a hungry cry from a cry due to a dirty or wet nappy. The myth that this information comes inherently to women is a serious mistake, however, and leaves many women who may not feel an immediate bond with their children, or who are not sure what to do, feeling very insecure and anxious.

As more and more women choose or are forced to work and men either choose to remain at home or have difficulty in finding work, roles are changing. Men may find themselves as the primary, or at least equal, carer for the new-born and the father finds himself to be the one who can best anticipate what the infant wants. It is sometimes helpful for the health visitor or midwife to explain to both parents that this knowledge comes from experience rather than from simply being either a mother or a father.

The 'Child as Ruler' myth

Another popular myth is that children are the most important resource for any society, and therefore anything that a child needs must come first. This myth is closely related to the one that states that parenting automatically involves sacrifice and that anyone who is not willing to sacrifice almost everything should not be a parent. While it may be true that children are important to a society, it must be firmly stated that parents are people, too. To be over-indulgent or to become a martyr to the child can cause as many problems as not paying enough attention to what that child needs. Trading one set of problems for another is not the goal of good parenting.

The 'Perfect Mother' myth

A well-known psychoanalyst and writer about child development named Donald Winnicott pointed out that what a child needs is 'good-enough mothering'. By this he meant that for healthy development a child needs to have its emotional and physical needs met often enough not to feel neglected or abandoned by the mother or mother-substitute. But he meant also that it is equally important that children learn how to cope with *not* having their needs met, too. In other words, the mother must be 'good enough', *not* perfect. An important part of becoming a mature human being is developing the ability to be able to wait, to consider the needs of others and to realize that even if mother does not come now, *this minute*, she will come in the end. Children whose needs are met every time they cry or demand something will never learn how to be tolerant, mature and sociable adults.

Debbie, a sensitive and very caring single parent, wanted her toddler Thomas to have everything he could possibly want without having to cry his heart out for it. He soon learned that if he wanted his mother to stop talking to a friend who had come to visit, or if he caught sight in a shop of a new toy that he fancied, all he had to do was to screw up his face and threaten to scream, and Debbie would do what he wanted. Thomas also learned that he could successfully stop his mother from spending much time with Mike, her boyfriend, by crying every time she paid attention to Mike. Debbie honestly thought she was doing a good job by being so responsive to Thomas, without realizing that she was allowing him to take over the household. She was failing to teach him about sharing and being considerate to others.

The 'Twenty-Four-Hour Mother' myth

Connected to the myth that parents should give up everything for their children is the idea that babies will be harmed if their mothers go out to work. This idea partly grew out of some research that was done by a psychiatrist called John Bowlby at the end of World War II. Bowlby studied young children who had been separated from their mothers and left in state nurseries and hospitals, with very little individual attention or emotional care. He noticed that these children were not only physically underdeveloped, but also emotionally deprived. They were withdrawn and sad, and he suggested that they were likely to grow up into emotionally crippled adults or delinquents.

Dr Bowlby's findings were then taken to mean that if children are separated from their mothers for any length of time, they will be harmed for life. As a result, women have been encouraged never to leave their children, and to abandon ideas of going back to work until the child had left school. Yet although Dr Bowlby was right to point out that children who are not given individual attention and love will lose an important part of normal and healthy growing up, he was mistaken in assuming that only mothers can provide this love and attention, or that mothers had to be there all day, every day. In fact, what a child does need is some love and physical contact from a person or a small group of people who want to spend time with that child. All children need mothering, but mothering can be provided by fathers, caring nannies, grandparents or friends, just as well as the mother. It is, however, important that the substitute mother does not chop and change. Plenty of recent studies have shown that nursery schools are fine for children so long as the quality of the care provided is good, and that children are treated as individuals. Modern thinking suggests that a working mother who spends a couple of happy hours at the end of a day with her child is better for that child than a full-time mother who is bitter and resentful about having to stay at home.

The 'Unimportant Father' myth

Connected to the 'twenty-four-hour-mother' myth is the myth that the father is not directly important to the bringing up of the child, but is only indirectly important by supporting and protecting the family. In the past it was sometimes assumed that the father had no direct bearing on the raising and the growth of the child, especially at the younger stages. This is shown to be obviously untrue as more and more fathers take a direct role in bringing up their children. But even in families where the father takes a more traditional role in providing the primary financial support for a family, he still plays a very important part in the development of a child. He is the model that the child, whether boy or girl, uses as the basis of what men can be expected to be like. Studies of families where there is no father present show that children without a father, or someone who fills the position of father, are more likely to have difficulties than those with a father present. In families with no father, a child is helped if someone from outside the immediate family, like a grandparent, teacher or boyfriend, supplies some of what is missing due to the absence of the father.

Fathers (or their substitutes) are often especially good at providing a different sort of play for the child, and in particular encouraging the child to take part in physically rough games. Such games are undoubtedly good for both boys and girls. Parents together show children what adult relationships are like, how to adapt to different demands of different people and how to share affection.

The 'Inheritance' myth

Another common myth is that parents who were raised poorly themselves will be 'bad' parents, and those that were raised 'correctly' will be 'good' ones. Although there are some links between the way parents are brought up and their own parenting style, this does not mean that just because someone was unhappily or badly brought up they will necessarily raise *their* children badly or unhappily. Nor does it mean that just because someone was brought up well they are immune from bringing up their children poorly. Humans are good at both learning and loving, and people do change. We all know someone who seems to have had an extremely deprived childhood and yet has developed into a kind and generous adult.

The 'Passive Adult' myth

The next myth is that the raising process is a learning experience only for the child, since the parents have already done their learning. The truth is that the child has almost as much effect on the parent as the parent has on the child. Any parent who has ever had a 'bad day' with their child will readily acknowledge this. How we feel, what we do and how we interact with the child is a direct result of how the child is feeling, what he or she is doing or how he or she is interacting with us. Yet many parents do not recognize the effect that their children have on them and see any learning along the way as confirmation that they are inadequate as parents. Because these parents do see a lack of knowledge as a negative statement about themselves, they will generally not tell the nurse that they do not know something which they think everyone else does. The challenge for the nurse is to help the parent to see that having a child is something that inevitably involves making mistakes, learning from those mistakes, and having lots of new experiences.

The 'Passive Child' myth

Perhaps even more exciting is the importance of realizing that even young babies are not simply passive beings for whom parents have to provide all the knowledge or stimulation. Babies are active explorers although in the early months they do not have very good control over their bodies or communication systems so they need a lot of help. Babies are not like empty cups with nothing in, which parents fill up while the child does nothing in return. In fact, even very small babies are surprisingly good at working out what is going on, because they respond to feelings and are actually able to have 'conversations' with their parents at a much younger age than we used to think. These are not conversations with words but are interactions without words where one of the 'speakers' is not very good at controlling legs, arms, smiles or cries, yet is nevertheless a powerful communicator. These interactions are crucial for early development.

Recent discoveries in child psychology have shown that the most responsive parents are those who interact with their babies by paying close attention to what the baby is 'saying'. For example, take the simple game of Peep-boh. In this game, adults have to notice where the child is looking and how the child is feeling if the game is to work properly. You may sometimes notice parents who have an extremely good sense of timing playing with their children, whilst there are others who are not really paying attention to the state of the child and who may play roughly when the child is sleepy or try to stop the game when the child is playful. This happens when the parent does not really see the child as a person who is part of an interaction. Instead, the game is played 'at' rather than 'with' the child. So it is important to see play as a 'conversation', not just as an adult 'doing' something to a child.

The 'Right Way To Do It All' myth

The final myth is that there is one particular 'right' way to bring up children. Every child is an individual and, as with adults, what might be right for one is not always the best for another. A popular song a number of years ago sang about 'different strokes for different folks', and the same thing can be said about children. Some babies are quiet and adjust easily to the demands of the adult world, quickly learn to sleep through the night and so on. Others are simply more restless and need more attention. Some children do not appear to enjoy being cuddled as much as others, and cannot be comforted by caresses and touch. There is no point in trying to impose what we think a child ought to want if the child clearly does not want it.

These differences can be most confusing to parents. For example, Martin and Gillian were non-identical twins, who were nevertheless treated almost identically by their parents. Yet while Martin was a peaceful, cuddly toddler, Gillian never seemed able to sit still, and nearly drove her mother to distraction by her constant tumbles and bumps. Furthermore, Gillian never seemed to want to cuddle for long. She was always up and away as soon as her mother would let her go. There was nothing wrong with either child, they simply had different dispositions.

PARENTING AND STEPCHILDREN

In the past, when people walked down the aisle to be married, they did so in the expectation that they were about to become deeply involved with one other person until death caused a parting. They would of course find that they had new relationships with members of the other person's family, but at least for a while there would be only the two of them.

Today, however, it is becoming more and more common to find people who are marrying for the second or third time, bringing children from one or more previous marriages. In the time that it takes to say 'I do', some people go from living alone to being the newest member of an already established family. If both partners have children it can be even more difficult for everyone to find their place in the new order of things.

The problems which are encountered by step-parents not only include all of those which natural parents have, but also involve some which are unique to step-parenting. Questions of discipline and methods of bringing up children are sometimes even more difficult to resolve when one of the parents has already established a particular style. Whilst one would expect that people who are contemplating entering a marriage involving stepchildren will have already discussed such matters, it may be that many do not. Even for those who have done so the difficulty of actually enforcing rules in practice is much more difficult than when talking about them in theory.

As noted in Chapter 6, new step-parents will often be on the receiving end of some hostility if they are seen as 'replacing' a natural parent. The step-parent may correctly or incorrectly be seen as the reason for breaking up the original family. Children often rebel against the authority of the new parent in these situations, and it takes everything that even the most skillful new parent can muster to retain the relationship when this happens. It can then be very important for the nurse to be aware of what is going on in the family.

Heidi was eight years old when her mother remarried after being divorced for two years. Shortly after the wedding Heidi's school performance, which had always been outstanding, began to decline, and she became more and more difficult to deal with at home. Her normally well-kept room began to look a shambles and she refused to do anything her parents asked until they got angry, shouting demands at the top of their voices. Often Heidi and her mother were reduced to tears while her step-father retreated into a sullen shell. After a couple of months in which this process became more and more common, Heidi's mother went to see her doctor complaining of headaches, and mentioned what was happening at home. A health visitor was asked to see Heidi.

Since both parents were very concerned and expressed a desire to have the family run smoothly again, the 'blame' for the family troubles seemed to rest solely with Heidi. After speaking with Heidi for a short while, the nurse began to realize that her behaviour was a result of how she felt about her new father, and her anger at her mother for letting a 'stranger' into the family. By explaining this to Heidi's parents and helping them to see how Heidi viewed the situation all three adults were able to sit down with Heidi and reassure her of her stability within the family. As the nurse visited again over the next few weeks, Heidi's behaviour changed and the family gradually settled down again.

Not all problems with step-parenting are problems of accepting a new person into the family, however. Some of the most difficult to deal with are those in which new parents find that while they may really love their new spouse, they really do not like their 'new' children. Alternatively, they may prefer their own children to those their new spouse had at the time of marriage.

John loved Maggie, his stepdaughter, very much. They got along well and spent a great deal of time together until the birth of Rachel. Rachel was John's first child and he was surprised at how strongly he felt about her. The more time he spent with baby Rachel the more guilty he felt about spending less time with Maggie. Because Maggie was his stepchild John felt he could not discuss the problem with his wife. It wasn't until a health visitor, on one of her normal visits, asked John if he felt differently about Rachel from how he did about Maggie that he was able to talk about it. Just the knowledge that what he felt was not unusual or a sign that he was a bad parent was enough for John to be able to relax and begin being with both Rachel and Maggie for themselves, each with their own individuality.

Often, however, step-parents may find themselves feeling even more compelled to do whatever is necessary and 'right' for their stepchildren than they would for their own children. It just seems a little more difficult to say no, rather like the child that you might babysit for. This can obviously lead to problems too, such as jealousy between children and resentment between parents or ex-spouses.

Looking at these feelings which are familiar to step-parents, it is easy to see that step-parenting has a lot of difficult problem areas over and above those that any parent might have. Not that there will automatically be problems. Many step-parents do get along well with their new family. If, however, problems do arise, some of the areas mentioned in this section might be possible causes.

PARENTING PROBLEMS WITH ADOPTED CHILDREN

There is one case in which parenting another's child is very similar to parenting one's own children, and that is in the case of adopted children. Being an adoptive parent differs from step-parenting in a number of significant ways:

- The child is 'chosen' prior to the adoption. In that sense the child is planned for rather than being an additional consideration.
- Both parents are, in most cases, actively involved in choosing the child.
- The child 'belongs' to both parents equally.

In these senses, the adopted child is very much like the natural child.

The difference, and most of the parenting problems, come from the fact that the child is not the biological child of the parents. In most cases there is the worry that some day the 'real' parents may want to see the child, or that when the child is old enough he or she will want to search for the real parents. While few parents attempt to contact their children who have been adopted, the vast majority of adopted children will sooner or later want some information about their natural parents, although most do not in fact try to trace them personally. But it is because of worries like this that problems sometimes arise, as the adoptive parents feel threatened or anxious that they might lose their adopted child emotionally, if not in fact.

Yet the evidence is that adoptive parents are in no way inferior to natural parents, and that adopted children love their adoptive parents as much as biologically related children do. There does not seem to be a need for a 'blood-bond' for parenting to be successful. Emotional bonds are the key issue. But the normal fears that most parents have that they may not have done a good job seem more worrying when the child is somehow 'not theirs'. As one adopting parent said, 'We have the best and the worst of both worlds. The best because we have the ability to choose the child we want and the worst because we can never say that we had no choice.'

The child's experience

One of the differences between adopted-parenting and step-parenting is that *both* parents are new to the child who is adopted or fostered. While there is one parent in a stepfamily who has been familiar to the child since birth, in an adopted family the child is a complete stranger to both parents. While this may not present too much difficulty for those who are adopted at a very young age, the older the child is at the time of adoption, the harder it can become.

For the child who is trying to fit into a new family the nature of the problem will depend on their age and whether or not the change is seen as permanent. Assuming that the child is old enough to be aware of the change, a number of things have to be coped with. Not only is there the loss of those who were familiar and who were depended upon at the child's last home, but there are new rules to be learned, different foods, different routines, and differences in what will be praised or discouraged. All of this occurs at a time when the new parents are likely to be nervous and somewhat uncertain themselves. Even though the parents may be told of the problems which might occur in these situations, they may still need reassurance and help at this early stage.

In her book *Adoption: A Second Chance*, Barbara Tizard notes that some of the most common problems with children who are adopted are temper tantrums, destructive behaviour and a lapse in toilet training. These may well occur as the child attempts to find out what the rules are in the new surroundings. 'How far I can go before I'm stopped, and will that remain the same for ever?' are questions that every child must ask in each situation. For those who are fostered, the questions arise and must be answered again each time they are placed in a new home.

PARENTING PROBLEMS WITH HANDICAPPED CHILDREN

We often assume that one of the most difficult situations in life must be to parent a handicapped child. It is difficult, but often not for the reasons which people usually imagine. In a survey of 50 children with physical handicaps, Dr Joan McMichael found that although 44 per cent of the children had slight or no emotional problems, 56 per cent of them had moderate or severe emotional difficulties in adjusting to their handicaps. The main symptoms included anxiety, depression, behaviour problems and temper tantrums. This is an important point to note because of the tendency of many people to focus on the physical problem and not pay attention to the emotional problems of children with handicaps. We have already made a similar point in Chapter 3.

All children want to be noticed and accepted, as do adults. We all like praise, and children are no exception. In a culture like ours, however, where many of our heroes are sports figures or film stars, and physical attractiveness is seen as particularly desirable, a child who is handicapped or disfigured can easily see the world as a place where he or she does not fit.

Parents, of course, may have difficulty with their children's handicap. As has already been noted, the guilt that often surrounds the birth of a handicapped child can be devastating. Questions of responsibility and self-recrimination are common, as is a tendency to try to find a cause, no matter how remote or irrational. While it may appear to be obvious that the parents did not have responsibility for the handicap, studies and surveys show that the vast majority of the parents of handicapped children at least initially feel some responsibility. In cases such as the Thalidomide disaster of the sixties the problem is even worse, since the parent, primarily the mother, sees the cause as having been of her own choosing. The child then may be seen as 'living proof' of the parent's mistake or poor judgement.

Whether the parent feels responsible or not there is still the problem of plans that had been made, or dreams that will be left unfulfilled. It is not uncommon for parents of 'normal' children to want their children to do things that they did not have the chance to do themselves, and when a physical or mental handicap prevents a child from fulfilling these parental wishes, all too commonly the parent sees it as a personal punishment. A consequence may be that the child is rejected. The primary task of a community nurse is to explore those feelings and to try to get the parents to re-evaluate them. Then the parents can get on with the task of providing what both they and the child need now, rather than regretting what may or may not have happened in the past or what may not happen in the future. Ask the parents to put into words their feelings about their present circumstances. Some of these feelings may be very irrational, and you should gently persuade the parents to examine them closely. Then you should try to steer the conversation towards planning for the present. You could try using the problem-solving approach that we described in the section on dialysis in Chapter 4.

A child's capabilities are often seen in comparison with others, and this too can form the basis for parental rejection. This is especially true in families where there are two or more children, one of whom is handicapped. Over time the handicapped child can be seen as both a 'nuisance', and, by virtue of the handicap, as less 'valuable' than the normal child. The consequences for the handicapped child can obviously be heart-breaking. The other possibility is that the parents will become over-protective and not allow the child to experience those things of which he or she *is* capable. Either of these responses by the parents can support and emphasize the 'different-ness' of the handicapped child. Again, the nurse who is aware of these possibilities and is willing to discuss them with either the parent or the child may well be on the way to helping a family overcome what might otherwise have been a considerable problem.

CONCLUDING REMARKS: PARENTS HAVE NEEDS TOO!

Earlier we said that children are people, but it is essential to remember that parents are people, too. As people, we all need time to ourselves, and that includes parents. It gives us the opportunity to recharge our batteries, explore new ideas, relax, or just consider alternatives before proceeding on a course of action. It is surprising how often parents (especially mothers) need reminding of this fact. Parents who never get a break from the process of parenting are doing a disservice not only to themselves, but also to their children.

In families where there are two parents willing to share the job of parenting, the opportunity to have personal time should arise easily. But in those families where there is only one parent, or where one parent is assigned the sole responsibility for parenting, it becomes more difficult. In such cases the ability to find time may involve additional costs, or increased demands on friends, at a time when there may be limited income and friends are busy with their own families. There are no easy answers to this problem, except that the nurse should try to support the single parent whenever possible, and try to encourage parents to share the child care as much as is feasible.

As we said at the start of this chapter, there are some occasions when parents do not consider their children's needs adequately, or when the process of caring breaks down completely. On some occasions, child abuse can result. This is the subject of the next chapter.

Suggestions for further reading

Bowlby, J. (1979) *Child Care and the Growth of Love*. London: Tavistock.
A classic text, which outlines Bowlby's ideas on child development and the need for love and attachment for healthy human personality growth. It should, however, be read in the light of the observations we have made in this chapter.

Dodson, F. (1970) *How to Parent*. London: Allen and Co.
   Numerous books have been written on how to be a good parent, but this one is short and reasonably priced. Of use to both nurses and parents, it discusses the subject of child development and gives practical advice in a clear-headed and jargon-free style.

Herbert, M. (1981) *Behavioural Treatment of Problem Children: A practical manual*. London: Academic Press.
   Nurses might well find this book useful when dealing with 'problem' children. It provides ideas for assessment and treatments and suggests ways of evaluating your efforts. It is, however, fairly advanced and is probably best seen as a very useful reference book.

Rutter, M. (1976) *Helping Troubled Children*. Harmondsworth: Penguin.
   Looks at some of the serious problems experienced in childhood and adolescence, and how they can be treated.

Chapter 9

When Things Go Wrong: The Problem of Child Abuse

No matter how experienced, emotions of disbelief, anger and amazement are felt by most professionals whenever they come across a case of child abuse. The idea that anyone could wilfully harm an innocent child is so disturbing that it is often difficult to believe it or work out why it has happened when you first suspect it. It is also difficult to accept that sometimes the most important thing to do is to report your suspicions rather than to 'protect' the family where you suspect it may be taking place. For nurses this can be especially difficult when most have entered the profession out of a strong desire to help, not to take on the role of family policeman. Yet community nurses will be among the first professionals to pick up cases of child abuse, and therefore carry a lot of responsibility for action. This responsibility, together with the distressing initial reactions which normally occur, may explain why dealing with child abuse is often listed as one of the chief areas of stress within nursing, and may well contribute to the onset of burnout (see Chapter 11).

WHAT IS CHILD ABUSE?

Child abuse involves actions consciously undertaken with reasonable knowledge that they will harm the child physically and emotionally. Reasonable knowledge means that a normal, reasonable person would see the actions as harmful. It is usually limited to acts which are carried out by those charged with the care of the child. Therefore, we will not in this chapter be looking at instances of cruelty to children who are harmed in the course of other crimes, such as robbery or kidnapping. Any father, mother, sister, brother, aunt, uncle, grandparent, live-in boyfriend or girlfriend, teacher or fosterparent can commit child abuse.

Sadly, we know it is fairly widespread and that it happens in families at all economic levels and all social classes.

Some people believe that child abuse is becoming more common nowadays, whilst others say that we are just hearing more about it than we used to. In practical terms it does not matter which view is right. What we do know is that it does exist and that every day many innocent children are suffering. In order to gain a perspective on child abuse and attempt to understand it, we can divide it somewhat arbitrarily into four basic types, and look at each one separately. These are: physical, sexual, and emotional abuse, and neglect.

PHYSICAL ABUSE

Physical abuse includes all of those instances in which an adult does some physical harm to a child by direct action. This includes hitting, striking, biting and burning. Of all the forms of abuse, physical abuse is the most easily detected since it leaves evidence – broken bones, bites, scars and bruises. It is also the most common form of abuse and has been recognized for the longest time. According to the NSPCC, physical abuse increased by 70 per cent between 1979 and 1984. In 1985 it was the assessed cause of six deaths and 93 serious injuries.

The first difficulty in reducing child abuse is to recognize it early. Question anything that just does not add up. An unusual number of accidents is a prime indicator. We all know that when children are small they tend to have a lot of bumps and falls: learning to walk is, in itself, a major feat. Those who have children have often winced as they imagine themselves suffering some of the falls that their children have while learning to walk. Children also tend to be very curious and, even with the most careful of parents, suffer from minor burns, cuts and abrasions. Few of us come through childhood totally unscathed.

However, a key difference between the normal child and the abused child is the frequency of those accidents. Even the most uncoordinated of children tend not to walk repeatedly into a door or fall down flights of steps. While the accounts of the 'accidents' may vary, you must be alert to the *possibility* of child abuse if something is said to have happened to account for the bruises and bumps almost every time you call in and, on detailed questioning, the account is oddly circumstantial and lacks appropriate detail.

There is a strong need to emphasize the word *possibility*. While most nurses may prefer to err on the side of safety (that is, reporting someone who is not abusing a child rather than overlooking one who is) it obviously does the nurse–patient relationship no good to accuse some-one of abusing their child when no such abuse exists. Although this may sound like a classic 'Catch 22', it really is not. It just means that the nurse must do all of the required 'homework' before reporting the case, though talking it through with a colleague may help to clear your mind about it.

Eddy was a beautiful blond-haired little boy with a round face. He was the image of a happy and wanted four-year-old boy. He was friendly and always had a smile when Kate, the health visitor, came to visit. It was very difficult for Kate to acknowledge the possibility of abuse when Eddy started to show multiple bruises each time she called in. Eddy's mother had always seemed to be a caring person, and although Eddy's father was away a great part of the time, he was not the type of person who would abuse a child, either.

After weeks of noting new bruises on each visit and hearing Eddy's mother explain them by saying that he had 'just bumped into a door' or 'he was just playing', Kate finally decided that Eddy was being abused. Fortunately, before Kate started the process of investigation by contacting the social services and arranging for Eddy to be placed on the 'at risk' register, she asked the general practitioner to carry out a full physical examination. The doctor took some blood samples, and had them tested. The results came back showing that Eddy was suffering from a severe case of aplastic anaemia. While they were discussing the results of the test and what treatment would be required in the future, Kate was able to tell Eddy's mother of her previous worries about the possibility of abuse, in such a way that Eddy's mother realized how much Kate cared about Eddy as an individual and not as 'just another patient'. During the remaining period of Eddy's treatment, Kate and Eddy's mother found that they could share many of Eddy's mother's fears and worries, and that the nurse–patient relationship had improved, not worsened.

On the other hand, if an error is going to be made, it is better to report a suspected case of child abuse that turns out not to be one than to let one go by that may be extremely serious. Just remember to check out the possibilities. Child abuse is like any other diagnosis that the team of health care professionals must make. You must have reasonable grounds for suggesting what you are diagnosing before you start investigating it in depth, otherwise you will cause a lot of unhappiness. In the absence of a good, sensible explanation you should investigate any cases of repeated bruising, broken bones or other signs of maltreatment.

Why does physical abuse occur?

The reasons for child abuse are many and varied. However, one point is important. Although some of the injuries inflicted on children are so dreadful that they are almost unbelievable, nevertheless, if we are honest, we can all probably admit to feeling aggressive towards our children at least once in our lives. Most of us know what it is like to feel desperate when trying to cope with a baby who, hour after hour, just will *not* stop crying. Equally, all parents know what it feels like to be infuriated by a toddler who keeps on and on asking the same questions, or whining or refusing to go to sleep.

However, it is also the case that most of us manage to control ourselves, so that we do not lash out at a child who is so much smaller and weaker than ourselves, realizing that the child is not deliberately behaving in this way just to annoy us. But those who do physically damage their children lose control. They often report feeling angry with the child, because the child is not 'behaving' well; that is, it is crying or refusing to eat. Of course, what they are saying is that the child is behaving like a child, but that they cannot cope with the demands this makes upon them to be tolerant and caring. Many child abusers are described as having very low 'frustration tolerance'. They cannot cope very well with the frustration of the child's 'misbehaviour' or continuing demands. Such low frustration tolerance can sometimes lead people to maltreat children in order to 'teach them a lesson' or to get them to 'behave properly'. In addition, abusers have difficulties establishing appropriate boundaries. By this we mean that they have difficulties deciding things like 'When does a spanking cease being a spanking and become a beating?' They simply cannot seem to work out when to stop.

In addition, researchers have found that people who abuse children are often unable to make relationships with adults in which they have to give as well as take. They see violence as the only way of getting what they want. People who are known to have committed physical abuse against a child describe feeling powerful at the time of the abuse, whereas in the rest of their lives they report feeling powerless and weak.

There is also a body of research that shows that many people who abuse children were abused themselves when they were children, but this is *not* always the case. Just because someone was abused as a child does *not* mean that they will abuse their own children; nor does it mean that only those who were abused as children will become abusers. We do know, however, that children who are abused tend to have difficulty establishing boundaries to what is appropriate in a given situation, and often have difficulties establishing and maintaining close personal relationships with other adults – the very things that are often found in people who abuse children.

SEXUAL ABUSE

Sexual abuse appears to be one of the fastest growing forms of child abuse, although here again it may be a result of more and better reporting of cases than a real increase in incidence, though it is more likely to be a combination of the two. From 1980 to 1984 sexual abuse rose from 1 per cent of all cases reported to the NSPCC to 11 per cent. In 1983, 51 cases were reported to the NSPCC, while there were 98 cases reported in 1984 and 222 in 1985. The highest risk group appears to be between the years of 10 and 14, just when children are approaching and experiencing puberty, although there were six cases reported in the 0–6 age group. In addition, some cases have been reported in the past with children as young as two months old.

Two facts about the sexual abuse of children are by now well established.

- Most victims of sexual abuse are girls. However, a survey at the University of California showed that almost 25 per cent of those who said that they had been abused as children were males, so it would be wrong to exclude boys from our discussion.

- Most people who commit abuse are male. In other words, the people who abuse both girls and boys are most likely to be males: their fathers, uncles, older brothers or others who are in the temporary position of parents, such as houseparents or teachers. Note though that some cases of sexual abuse by females do take place, so the possibility of abuse by women must not be overlooked.

The nature of the abuse varies. It may take the form of asking the child to watch certain acts, or the child may be asked to fondle the genitals of the adult. Alternatively, the adult may attempt to touch the child in a sexually intimate way. In some cases, the child may be coerced into sexual intercourse with the adult.

Discovering sexual abuse

Because of its highly personal nature, sexual abuse is particularly difficult to uncover. Few victims of sexual abuse are willing to disclose it until long after it has happened. Not only is there an invasion of the body and all the complicated physical and emotional problems which go along with that, but there may well be additional feelings of guilt or responsibility. Not only are sexually abused children likely to feel as though they have caused or created the situation, but they may also be faced with protecting both the abuser and the family as a whole. Other victims are told that if they disclose the abuse they will not be believed, will cause the abuser to be sent to prison, will cause the breakup of the family or will be sent away themselves. It is also common for the perpetrator to suggest or state outright that as long as the victim remains 'willing' and quiet, brothers or sisters will be 'spared', although this is rarely the case in fact.

Sexual abuse tends to start as a 'private' relationship between the abuser and the victim. The victim is often told that he or she is special and that what is happening is something that cannot be shared with anyone else in the family, and that in fact the others would not understand anyway. Because of the idea that they are in some way special and have access to a 'privileged' relationship with the abuser, and also because they may be threatened by the abuser, victims are often in a position where the disclosure of the abuse is more threatening than the abuse itself.

Since it is often almost impossible for victims to report directly that they are being abused, it becomes even more important for adults to be sensitive to clues which might indicate possible abuse. One of the first clues that sexual abuse could be going on is an inappropriate level of power held by the child within the family. If a parent has started an incestuous relationship with one or more of the children, then the other parent has literally been replaced. This may well lead to a situation in which it becomes too threatening for the replaced parent to 'see' what is happening within the family. Now, not all children who exercise power within a family are the victims of child sexual abuse, but if a daughter has obviously replaced her mother as the primary female or a son his father as the primary male, there must be a reason. Sexual abuse is at least a possibility.

Another clue is an unusual degree of sexual awareness or behaviour on the part of the child. This can happen if a child is taught to relate to adults, or members of the opposite sex in general, through sexual means. It can also happen if love and sex have become virtually interchangeable, as they so often have for victims of sexual abuse. Again, while there might be other reasons for such 'promiscuity', the possibility of sexual abuse should not be ignored.

Jeannie, a pretty little six-year-old, enjoyed painting at her school, and always chose to spend time at the easel during play periods. One day she presented her teacher with a picture of a man with a very large and obviously erect penis. Jeannie's teacher, although rather shocked by the picture, was sensitive enough to take Jeannie on one side and ask her about the picture. This gave Jeannie the chance to tell her teacher about some of the things that were going on at home while her mother was out at work, and which she was too frightened to tell anyone else. The teacher's sensitivity to Jeannie's apparent promiscuity meant that the sexual abuse that she was suffering at the hands of her father could be dealt with. If Jeannie's teacher had simply scolded the little girl for an obscene painting the problem would never have been discovered.

Along with an increased sexual awareness comes a change in the natural pattern of relationships in general. A young woman who has been involved in a sexual relationship with someone since the age of seven or eight can hardly be expected to share the interests of most 13 or 14-year-olds who begin to notice boys and start dating. In a sense the child has been robbed of his or her childhood. As one victim stated, 'What's the point in playing the game when you've already won the prize?' But in child sexual abuse, the child *is* the prize, and wins little or nothing for himself or herself. Instead, a sad and bewildered maturity will signal the destruction of childhood in such victims.

Who is the sexual abuser?

In working with sexual abusers, as with physical abusers, some observations are made again and again. For example, abusers report feeling a sense of power during the abuse. As one abuser said, 'Even if I can control nothing else in my life, when I'm with her she's doing what I want her to do. I'm in control.' The paradox that escapes most abusers is that once sexual abuse has occurred, the child has a secret which most abusers find extremely threatening. In order to keep the child quiet, they may well resort to bribery or terror.

As was noted with physical abusers, sexual abusers often have a difficulty in establishing appropriate boundaries. When the natural affection of a child is used for sexual purposes by an adult then boundaries have been confused and crossed. Obviously, and according to the law, the primary responsibility to set limits lies with the adult and not with the child. Child sexual abusers, however, seldom see it this way, and may defend themselves by saying things like, 'But she liked it! In fact, she used to dress seductively in order to make me do it!' Yet this overlooks the fact that adults are supposed to be able to make decisions about what is right and what is wrong, and to take care of children, not to exploit them for their own pleasure. The law makes it clear that the adult is responsible in all such cases.

What are the effects of sexual abuse?

Unlike physical abuse, there are few easily observable bruises and cuts to heal. Most of the damage takes place at the emotional level. As with all child abuse, victims often have problems when they grow up in establishing and maintaining relationships. They may have difficulties in trusting others, especially people who resemble the abuser. In every developed culture, adults are held responsible for children and have restrictions placed on them to govern their behaviour towards children. Even in those cultures that allow what we might consider to be, effectively, incest (like brothers being able to have sex with each others' wives) the person who takes responsibility for raising children is forbidden to have any sexual relationship with them. This allows at least one 'safe' relationship for the child in which he or she can develop and feel love without the risk of exploitation. In this safe relationship, the child can test behaviours and find out what is appropriate and what is not. The breaking of this basic trusting relationship makes it hard for the child to establish a basic trust in any subsequent relationship. 'How can I trust another man when I couldn't even trust my own father?' has been heard in various forms from many victims of sexual abuse. Hence it is that problems with relationships are one of the main results of abuse. If the trust which underlies all relationships has been eroded or destroyed, then a future relationship itself can mirror that lost trust.

Mrs Miles, 25, had been sexually abused from the age of three until her father left home when she was six. At the time Mrs Miles came to the attention of the nursing service she was married and had a daughter, Tracy, who was three years old. A nurse was asked by the family doctor to visit the home to check on Tracy, who had been inexplicably ill for about two months. The illness was never serious enough to require Tracy to be admitted to a hospital, but it was serious enough to keep her from being able to get out and play, and seemed to prevent attendance at the surgery.

When talking with Mrs Miles, the nurse noticed that it was difficult to distinguish when Mrs Miles was talking about her own father, and when she was talking about her husband, Tracy's father. They were always described in the same way. Having had some experience with child sexual abuse, the nurse became alerted when Mrs Miles mentioned that she would not let her husband care for Tracy and then refused to give a reason for her decision. By talking to Mrs Miles the nurse also discovered that she would not let Tracy sleep in her bedroom alone. On several occasions, Mrs Miles commented that if Tracy was in hospital she would be 'safe'. However, there was no physical evidence that Tracy was in fact being abused. It was simply that Tracy never seemed to be very healthy, and was always suffering from one minor complaint after another.

After a while the nurse managed to persuade Mrs Miles to go on her own to see her family doctor, who eventually discovered the root of the problem. It turned out that when Tracy had reached the age of three, Mrs Miles had thought it 'safer' for her daughter to be sick than to have to undergo the abuse that she herself had suffered as a child at that age. In a sense, Mrs Miles was keeping her daughter sick in order to 'protect' her. Although there was no evidence that Mr Miles would abuse Tracy, Mrs Miles had been too frightened to trust him, because, after all, she had trusted her own father, and look what had happened to her.

Mrs Miles' case underlines the not uncommon fact that some people will take a great deal of time to overcome the effects of child abuse. While it may well be outside the responsibilities of nurses to treat such longstanding problems, they can be instrumental in discovering not only current child abuse but also victims of past experience who are still living under its effects. They will therefore be able to initiate effective action.

EMOTIONAL ABUSE

Of all forms of abuse, emotional abuse is the hardest to detect and probably the most difficult to put right. There are no visible scars as in physical abuse and no single event which can be focused upon and prevented as in sexual abuse. In fact those who have been emotionally abused are often the very type of children who would generally be least noticeable in a crowd. They are often quiet, withdrawn or exceptionally 'good', and frequently go unrecognized as a consequence.

Another reason why emotional abuse is so difficult to recognize is that it is a process which many of us have experienced at some time or another, both as abusers and victims, even if it was not very damaging in the long run. It occurs when we make unwarranted or unsupported hurtful comments about someone else. Part of the problem is that while such comments or insults are abusive they are not always intended to be hurtful. For example, a number of comedians have made a very good living by insulting their audiences, much to the delight of those being insulted. But it is when the person being spoken to believes that the person speaking really *means* what is being said that abuse takes place. It is very difficult for young children *not* to believe what is said by adults. After all, adults do seem to know everything. If parents, in the eyes of a child, know all and see all, it is easy to believe that what they say must be right, including all their hurtful comments.

Another form of emotional abuse happens when adults repeatedly make things that should be readily available to children conditional. While comments like, 'If you don't eat all of your parsnips, you won't get any trifle', may not be abusive, statements such as, 'If you don't do as you're told, I won't love you any more' and, 'I'll leave you behind if you cry when the doctor gives you the injection' ·probably are. No child should have their own worth and lovableness continually put to the test like this. If children are 'bribed' like this, they soon come to believe that, indeed, they are not worthy of love, and they are in fact not good people. To feel that you have to do exactly what your parents want in order to be loved is obviously not a very happy start to life, and is unlikely to create feelings of self-confidence as you grow older.

Equally cruel is making children feel responsible for things over which no normal person has control, or where the child cannot possibly be to blame. This sometimes happens when parents are under a lot of stress, but even so, the consequences for the child can be very distressing. For example, the child can be blamed for a family tragedy, totally unjustly, and can go through life feeling guilty in consequence. The comment 'If you hadn't said you hated your brother, he wouldn't be dying now' was actually heard on a children's cancer ward. That is not a recipe for the child's healthy psychological development.

Emotional abuse also tends to set up what is called a 'self-fulfilling prophecy'. If children are told that they are stupid often enough, they will tend to develop difficulties in learning which are not simply due to a lack of intelligence. After all, children are very easily convinced of all sorts of things. Think of all the children who believe that there really is a man who rides in a flying sleigh, pulled by eight reindeer each Christmas! Imagine a child who grows up hearing daily comments like, 'Idiot! You *are* stupid!', or 'You can't do anything right, can you?' It is surprisingly easy to convince children that they are worthless, stupid and unwanted.

Because of the problems that we have noted already the recognition of and professional response to emotional abuse has been somewhat limited in the past. The records do not go back very far, since the NSPCC state that they did not monitor emotional abuse before 1980. We do know, however, that there were 22 cases of emotional abuse reported to the NSPCC in 1985 and that this is most likely to be only a small proportion of those occurring.

Who are the emotional abusers?

Adults who are prone to practise emotional abuse have some characteristics in common. Most have unrealistic expectations of children's capabilities. In addition they also tend to believe that a child's behaviour is a direct reflection of their own worth as people, as well as their ability as parents. When these two ideas are put together the child may well suffer. For example, if children are expected to excel at some particular sport although they might not actually like it, and if their parents see the children's inability to excel as saying something bad about them as parents and as people, then the parents may well blame the child for any lack of success. This means that it was the children's fault, not the parents'. Unfortunately, children normally accept the blame from adults, who are of course much 'wiser' than they are.

Another typical instance of emotional abuse happens when a child becomes linked with some bad past experience through no fault of the child. An example of this might be a woman who has become pregnant just prior to a very traumatic divorce and has decided to keep the child only to find after the child is born that the mere sight of the child reminds her of her awful husband. It is sometimes hard to love something that reminds you of bad times, and people who would normally not be abusers can find themselves reacting in emotionally abusing ways. Clearly, the past is not the child's fault, yet it is the child who will suffer.

NEGLECT

'But I haven't done anything to my child!' is a plaintive cry heard by many people who have worked with child neglect cases. For some reason those who neglect their children believe that to harm a child one must 'do something' to them. The idea that doing nothing or not doing anything might harm a child is completely foreign to them. Unfortunately, this is far from the truth.

The work of the psychologist Harry Harlow is relevant here. He took some baby monkeys and divided them into three groups. Some he left with their mothers; some he put with soft, cuddly 'toys' to act as mother replacements; and some he put with just a wire feeding holder. What he found was that those who remained with their mothers developed at a normal rate. Those who were with soft, cuddly replacements were more withdrawn, and when put in with other monkeys interacted with them rather poorly. But the baby monkeys that were put in with the wire feeders were *very* withdrawn, isolated and would avoid interactions with other monkeys when given the chance.

Human babies tend to develop in similar ways when it comes to learning how to interact with others. Those who have warm, caring relationships with other family members tend to grow easily into healthy caring adults. Those who do not have more difficulty in developing relationships. Those who are completely isolated have a very difficult time indeed. Musicians and poets have long repeated the theme 'I want to be loved by you'. We all need others to love and be loved by if we are to develop into normal, happy human beings. If we do not receive some contact with or feedback from others we will not develop fully. This is where neglect enters the picture. Whether wilful or not, the withholding of attention and affection from children can cause a retardation in their development into mature, sensitive adults.

We have all heard tragic stories about children who have been locked in cupboards, bedrooms or worse, but neglect includes more than just the starvation or abandoning of a child. Any behaviour that neglects the needs of the child, emotional or physical, is neglect. Neglecting parents are often unaware of or unconcerned by the needs of their children, so that the child is not treated as a human being who has appropriate rights or even feelings.

As with emotional abuse, there are insufficient records to monitor the extent of neglect over a long period of time. Because of this we cannot be certain of general trends. However, they appear to be similar to the figures for emotional abuse in that they tend to fluctuate from year to year. We do know that both neglect and emotional abuse tend to occur with younger children rather than adolescents, since by the time children become adolescents they have usually developed defensive ways of safeguarding themselves.

Failure to thrive

One special category of neglect is failure to thrive. It has many of the hallmarks of neglect, but differs in a few important ways. First of all failure to thrive may well stem from organic or biological causes. Because of this it is very important for any nurse suspecting failure to thrive to ensure that any necessary homework has been done. For example, there are some children who may have difficulty digesting specific forms of fat or protein. In these cases the parent can be competent and caring, yet the child still becomes more and more malnourished.

The second difference between neglect and failure to thrive is that most agencies define failure to thrive as occurring only between birth and three years old. After that it is generally classed as a case of neglect. The age rule is not hard and fast, but is generally considered as a defining line, since most children either have or have not been thriving by the age of three. In addition, since children develop more quickly within the first three years, any lack of development is more apparent at this time and therefore failure to thrive is generally more easily noticed.

If we rule out any medical cause for a failure to thrive and just look at the non-medical causes we note that there is little difference between what causes neglect and what causes a failure to thrive. In discussing neglect we spoke of the tendency for the abusers to be either unconcerned or unaware of the needs of the children and the same process tends to occur in cases of failure to thrive.

In such cases it helps if the nurse is also aware of the emotional state of the parents. It may be difficult for parents to be aware of what their children need when they are involved with trying to get what *they* feel *they* need. This is especially true if their wants or desires are in conflict with their children's needs or desires.

Jackie was a young mother, recently divorced. She found herself alone and lonely and decided to start getting out more. Since she had married her school boyfriend she had not dated many people and decided that now was a good time to widen her horizons. Although she normally had someone look after her child while she was out, if she expected to be gone for only an hour or so she would often leave the child alone asleep in her cot. As babysitters were rather expensive she soon gave up bothering to arrange to have someone in, even if she expected to be out for the whole evening. Sometimes she would meet someone at a discotheque, and would ask him home to spend the night with her. Often the two of them would have quite a lot to drink, and Jackie sometimes realized she'd forgotten all about the baby until the morning.

It wasn't that Jackie didn't love her baby or that she wanted to hurt her, she was just so concerned about trying to end her own loneliness that she failed to realize that the baby also needed her time and affection. The situation was finally brought to light by a health visitor, who noticed that Jackie's child was only 24 inches tall and weighed only 24 pounds at the age of two years. After all medical causes were ruled out, Jackie was introduced to a group of other young single mothers. They met once a week with a counsellor and were able to talk about the problems they had with trying to run a family and still function as young women. As Jackie learned how others felt, and that she was not the only person to feel the way she did, she began to become more aware of what the baby needed. Within a year the baby was as tall and heavy as most three year olds and Jackie was much happier with both herself and her relationship with her daughter.

Of course, since no parents can be totally responsive to all their children's needs at all times, we have all probably experienced some form of 'neglect' either as children or as parents, at some time or another, even if it was only very minor. Indeed, as we suggested in Chapter 8, one important part of growing up is learning to cope with the absence of your parents, and being able to tolerate *not* having all your needs met immediately. But as with all other forms of child abuse, neglect becomes abuse when the welfare of the child is at stake. It is often up to community nurses to discover whether neglect might be taking place, and to decide whether it should be reported. Sometimes such a decision is very difficult to reach, and the support of your colleagues can be extremely important. Do not hesitate to get a second opinion, if there is any chance of a case of neglect having taken place.

FINAL COMMENTS

Throughout this chapter we have tried to suggest some of the problems of dealing with child abuse. Of all the issues that we have noted, however, none is as difficult for most people as the problem of deciding whether or not to report a case. This becomes particularly difficult for a nurse who has been trained to help people rather than to 'police' them. Since the last thing any nurse wants to do is to alienate the very people for whom help is intended, such decisions are very difficult. The best advice which we can give is that if after all considerations are taken into account there is still a question, then report it. It is easier to explain to an angry adult why you did report a questionable situation than to explain to an injured or dead child why you did not.

Suggestions for further reading

CIBA Foundation (1984) *Child Sexual Abuse within the Family*. London: Tavistock.
A handbook providing guidance on the types of actions which should be taken by professionals who encounter a case of child sexual abuse. Straightforward and helpful in its approach.

Jones, D.N. (ed.) (1982) *Understanding Child Abuse*. London: Hodder and Stoughton.
Provides an overview of the problem of child abuse, together with practical advice concerning its recognition and treatment. It is both reasonably priced and readable.

Kelly, J.A. (1983) *Treating Abusive Families*. London: Plenum Press.
Fairly academic in approach; provides an outline of some of the types of treatment available for abusing families. Concentrates primarily on cases of physical abuse.

Kempe, R. and Kempe, E. (1978) *Child Abuse*. London: Fontana/Open Books.
Probably the best-known overview of child abuse in all its manifestations. It includes a comprehensive discussion of treatments available and prevention.

Chapter 10

Stress and the Nurse: A Daily Encounter

Open any magazine or newspaper and it seems as if everyone is talking about stress. Schoolchildren taking exams are said to be suffering from it; train drivers are, too; Members of Parliament are stressed; policemen are stressed; even tax inspectors are said to be stressed! Research on stress in hospitals has shown that patients suffering cardiac arrest or diabetes are made worse by stress, whilst relatives of the mentally ill are advised to make the sufferer's life as free from stress as possible.

For nurses, stress has the status of an occupational hazard. For patients, stress is an added complication to illness. But why should nurses and their patients feel so stressed?

NURSES, PATIENTS AND STRESS

Firstly, the stresses experienced by nurses relate directly to the task of nursing. The daily task of the nurse is to interact with someone who is in need, or in pain, and to deal with that person in a way that makes them feel better, happier or more comfortable. Yet as Henry Stack Sullivan, a psychotherapist, once said:

> Interaction with significant people constitutes the most difficult sort of action required of us. People are decidedly the hardest thing we have to deal with.

Patients are the significant people who define a nurse's professional functions, but they do not usually come when they are feeling good, to give cheer, or to congratulate, compliment or encourage. They come with their fears, pains and doubts, seeking help. And that is where the stresses start for nurses.

128

Secondly, for patients, the sources of stress may be different in that they are worried about their illness, their families and their future. As every nurse knows, being stressed makes the process of recovery much slower, and in some cases may even have brought the condition on in the first place.

All of this means that the cost of stress in both financial and personal terms is enormous. So what is stress? How does it affect patients? And how does it affect nurses? This chapter explores the nature of stress, what it is and how it can be handled, in nurses themselves and in their patients. The next chapter looks in more detail at some of the consequences for the nursing profession of *not* paying attention to stress.

WHAT IS STRESS?

Perhaps the best place to start is with the physical sensations that we all experience when feeling under pressure. These are the biological responses to stress which occur in three stages.

The first stage, originally described by a physiologist named Hans Selye, is the coping response of a person or animal to some threatening situation. Selye pointed out that the stress response happens when a person or animal starts to adapt to threat. The individual reacts by either trying to escape from what is stressful. ('flight') or trying to deal with it aggressively ('fight'). That is fine when the threat in question is something that can be run away from (like the attack of a larger animal), or can be fought (like an enemy); but when the threat is something like an examination or an interview, neither flight or fight is a very helpful response. Unfortunately, the fact that a threat may be real or merely perceived makes no difference. If an examination or interview is seen as a threat to your achievement of a desired goal, the body's reaction to it will be real.

The physiological reaction to stress includes the following:

1. *Pupil dilation and extended peripheral vision.* (To help you perceive the danger more readily.)

2. *Increased muscle tension.* (You feel yourself jump or tremble.)

3. *Increased breathing rate.* (You breathe more rapidly and superficially.)

4. *Vaso-constriction.* (The blood vessels in your fingers and toes constrict to push the blood back to the central part of your body where it is most needed – your fingers and toes get cold, which may be the origin of the term 'cold feet' when someone is scared.)

5. *Increased heart rate.* (You can feel your heart thumping, and if it is bad enough, you may fear – incorrectly – that you are having a heart attack.)

6. *Gastro-intestinal changes.* (You may want to pass water frequently, vomit, or have diarrhoea.)

7. *Adrenalin discharge.* (Experienced as having butterflies in the stomach.)

8. *Decreased muscle tone.* (You feel weak or trembling.)

Stages and symptoms of stress

The symptoms described occur in the first stage. Most of us have experienced some or all of these sensations at times of high stress, such as taking a driving test, going for an interview, or before having a difficult conversation with someone who is important to us.

If the threat continues over a period of time, and the attempts to cope with it have not been successful, the second stage of the stress response will occur. Here the person continues to try to resist the stress, but some organic changes start to take place in the body. The continuing increase in heart rate can lead to high blood pressure, and the gastrointestinal changes may lead to stomach ulcers or colitis. The person under stress may at this stage not even realize that these physical changes are taking place. For example, chronic bad relationships at work can be very stressful and may lead to these physical changes without the individual even noticing.

The final stage of stress is reached when attempts to cope with the threat have failed and resources are nearly exhausted. At this point physical catastrophe can occur, such as a heart attack. Some people may withdraw completely from interacting with friends and family through depression. Yet others may experience a 'delayed shock' reaction, in which they constantly relive the stress-provoking problems of the past. This can be particularly difficult for the family, as well as for the individual. Traumatic memories or dreams may haunt the patient, who will be very difficult to help or comfort. Eventually death may occur, although the final cause of death may be some apparently unrelated illness or condition.

Of course, people who are under stress feel not only physical symptoms but also psychological ones. They feel panicky and upset, unable to concentrate, they may forget things, and appear to others preoccupied or jumpy. Inside, the sense is of being unable to cope, and that everything is just beyond them. The simple tasks they are having to deal with appear too difficult, or there is simply too much to be coped with all at once. Psychologists have seen this as the most important aspect of stress: the gap or imbalance between what a person sees as being demanded of them, and their diminished ability to meet those demands. This imbalance is typically invisible to anyone except the person feeling the stress. Thus an important part of the actual state of being stressed is how each person perceives what is being demanded, and the extent of his or her own resources to meet those demands.

WHAT CAUSES STRESS?

Because an important part of being stressed is the imbalance between what is seen as the problem and the estimate of what can be done about it, it follows that what may be stressful for you will not necessarily be stressful for me: it depends on how we each see things, and what we think our own abilities are. For example, I might find the idea of spending the whole afternoon alone with three lively toddlers extremely stressful, while standing up and lecturing to a class of students would be no problem. You might find the exact opposite to be true for you. But both of us would feel equally stressed, me in the playroom, and you in the classroom. In addition, stress takes different forms for different people. Some people have physical symptoms like butterflies in the stomach, while others find they are getting irritable and tired all of the time.

Stress at work

People often say that work is 'stressful'. But the way in which it is stressful and the reason why it is stressful also differ between people. Some people are stressed because they have too much to do, and others feel stressed because they have too little to do. Research psychologists have shown that some of the most stressed members of the work force are not managers and top executives working apparently under great pressure but assembly line workers who are stressed by not having enough to do, or having routine, boring jobs to do, or feeling that they have no influence over what they do. It has also been found that some of the most stressed members of society are the unemployed, who probably have the least to do. So stress depends on the individual's own view of the situation and his or her judgement of what is needed to cope with it.

   Stress can be experienced quickly, as when you suddenly realize that a member of the family that you are visiting is getting extremely angry and appears to be threatening violence, or it can develop slowly. In the first case, the physical reactions you experience (heart beating fast, sweating hands, dry throat) can be felt immediately, and will usually subside again when you leave the stressful situation (although you may feel panicky again when you think about it later on that day). But when stress comes on slowly it is rarely easy to pinpoint the exact cause. The physical symptoms may be less obvious, and will probably last longer.

Pauline was an experienced community nurse, with plenty of energy and enthusiasm for her work. She had a regular group of patients on one housing estate whom she visited every week to give routine injections to. When one of her colleagues went on maternity leave, she offered to take over the care of one or two additional cases on the estate who were known to be particularly difficult. At the same time, her own elderly mother became ill, and Pauline felt she ought to spend as much time as possible with her.

Pauline was becoming physically tired, but was coping reasonably well until a violent incident took place on the estate. This involved the child of one of the families that she had taken over from her colleague. Pauline felt she had to be even more vigilant than before, and although she wasn't spending any more time on the estate, found she was thinking about the family at home in the evenings, and was having difficulty sleeping. She noticed that when she woke up in the mornings she was feeling irritable and anxious and felt rather sick most of the time. She began to fear that she would no longer be able to do her job properly.

When Pauline contacted her senior at work for advice she was told that her department had every confidence in her ability to handle the situation. Yet Pauline didn't feel she was handling the situation at all well, and was beginning to worry that she could herself be sickening for something serious. None of the events that had occurred seemed to be enough to cause her to panic, and the advice from her senior made her feel that she had no reason to worry. She went to see her doctor, who told her to take two weeks off work because of 'nervous exhaustion'.

As is so often the case, the stress that Pauline experienced was caused by a combination of smaller events, which by themselves wouldn't have been much of a problem. Reassurance had not helped because it did not take account of what Pauline herself felt about the situation. On the contrary, it added to it since it made her feel as though she should be coping and wasn't; another example of a gap between what was required of her and what she was able to give.

Stress at home

Of course stress is not limited to work; our personal, private lives can be stressful, too. After all, it is usually our private lives that bring us most of our pleasures and sorrows, so perhaps it is not surprising if we sometimes find our personal lives more of a strain than our working lives. Perhaps the most difficult thing which Pauline had to cope with was the illness of her elderly mother, rather than the demands made by her patients. Like the relatives of many of her patients, Pauline was becoming both physically and emotionally exhausted by having to look after someone that she loved. Her emotional involvement with her own mother made this more stressful for her than her contact with the elderly people she saw regularly as part of her job.

There are a number of different sources of stress in our personal lives. Psychologists have found that a person can become stressed when *any* changes in the family take place, even if these appear to be welcome. Change has to be adapted to, and this can in itself be stressful. A new job, a birth in the family, marriage or a major change in routine can all be stressful as well as happy experiences. With big changes a person has to learn new ways of behaving and this can be a source of difficulty.

Steve had been looking forward to living with Wendy for many months before they finally found a suitable flat and could move in together. He had eagerly anticipated their being able to spend time on their own together, and had enjoyed planning how they would arrange their flat and belongings. When they eventually did move house, however, he found himself feeling irritable and unaccountably depressed, despite feeling still as much in love with Wendy as before. After a few weeks these feelings lifted, as he grew accustomed to having someone else around all of the time. The change in his living arrangements had been much more stressful than he had imagined, despite being exactly what he had wanted. So change of any sort, no matter how positive, can still be stressful.

More typically, however, people experience stress as a result of unpleasant experiences occurring either suddenly or gradually. A marriage in which there is little or no communication, poor housing, unemployment, poverty, or chronic sickness are commonly associated with feelings of stress, but the people that a community nurse visits may be stressed from a variety of sources. What is water off a duck's back to one patient may be extremely unpleasant to another. For instance, a referral for a gynaecological examination may be terrifying for some patients but not for others. The community nurse has to be extremely sensitive to the individual needs of each patient. Do not assume that just because you would not find something unpleasant your patient will not either. It is easy for health professionals to forget that hospitals are frightening and stressful places to people who are not used to them.

The stress of unemployment

The stress of unemployment has received a lot of attention in recent years. A number of studies have shown that people who are made redundant are at risk of becoming depressed, irritable and frustrated. If unemployment continues they seem gradually to lose their determination to get involved in life. Although on the face of it they might seem to have more time than the employed to get involved in leisure activities, such as sport, hobbies and voluntary work, they actually do less of these things than employed people. Financial worries and family pressures make the situation worse, especially as wives are more likely to be out of work if their husbands are also out of work. On the other hand when a wife *is* at work and the husband is not this can lead to feelings of inadequacy in the man, especially if he has been brought up in a rather rigid and stereotyped way to think that he is not a 'proper man' unless he is working. However, unemployment is not any easier for women: a number of studies have shown that it is girls, not boys, who are most badly affected by being unemployed.

Unemployment undoubtedly has an adverse effect on a person's mental health. Figures have shown that a rise in unemployment is linked to an increase in the suicide rate. Nevertheless, as we have said, individuals differ in their responses to stress. There is some evidence that for a minority of people, being unemployed is actually good for their mental health.

The stress of bad news

Some situations are likely to be stressful to almost anyone. The birth of a handicapped child or a stillbirth is an intensely distressing and difficult experience. It not only brings grief and a sense of disappointment but also worries such as 'What will happen now?'; 'Will I ever be able to have a normal baby?'; 'Was it my fault?' In these situations it is safe to assume that the level of stress as well as distress of all parents will be very high. Other situations which are known to be very stressful include the diagnosis of a serious or fatal illness, such as cancer or heart disease. Coming to terms with bad news may mean altering all the plans and hopes for the future. Such changes could not but be stressful.

The stress of caring

As we have already observed, some stresses develop slowly and the pressures increase gradually and are made worse if little relief or change seems possible. Providing constant care for an elderly, highly dependent and dementing relative is one such situation. Numerous studies have shown that the carers for the elderly suffer from a lot of the physical and psychological symptoms of stress. Although devoted to the old person, and determined not to allow them to be hospitalized, the carer (who is most likely to be the dementing person's spouse, or may be a son or daughter) may, not surprisingly, begin to feel worn out and resentful that a person who now appears to be almost a stranger is requiring so much time and energy.

When Sandra's mother became gradually less able to look after herself, Sandra and her husband Paul asked her to move in to live with them. Sandra had always been very close to her mother, and felt a great deal of loyalty to her, especially as her mother had been a great support when Sandra's first marriage had broken up. At first the problems didn't seem to be too great, as the dementia was not very far advanced. However, as the months passed, Sandra found that her mother often failed to recognize her, and had for some reason become extremely frightened of Paul. This meant that Sandra's mother would not allow Paul to assist in any way, leaving all the lifting and heavy work to Sandra. Consequently Sandra became extremely tired, whilst Paul was unable to help in any substantial way. Sandra felt unable to leave her mother alone in the house, as she had started wandering. Arguments began to flare up between Sandra and Paul. Sandra accused Paul of not helping, despite knowing that this was not his fault, while Paul said that, after all, it was not his mother. The community nurse, who was calling regularly to bath Sandra's mother, found she was spending most of her time listening to Sandra's worries. Feeling she would be letting her mother down, Sandra refused all offers of some respite care, although she did accept that she was getting more and more impatient with her mother. It was only when the community nurse gently pointed out that Paul too was at the end of his tether that Sandra admitted that she was under stress, and did need a break.

> *Sandra had felt that it was somehow wrong for her to feel stressed, in the belief that this implied she no longer loved her mother. The community nurse helped Sandra to see that the situation she was in was a stressful one, and that to feel stressed was neither wrong nor disloyal. In fact Sandra eventually agreed that to do something to reduce her own level of stress, by having a break from caring for her mother, might be the very best thing she could do for everyone, including her mother.*

All of the research that has been done on caring for the elderly or severely mentally or physically handicapped suggests that whatever the positive aspects, having constantly to attend to someone who is unlikely to improve is exhausting, both physically and emotionally. Nurses have a crucial role to play here in caring for the carers.

The stress of not knowing

The unknown can create fear. People become stressed not only because they do not think they have the ability to cope with a situation, but also because they do not know what to expect. If you cannot make sense of what is happening, then it is not surprising if you feel out of control and in a panic. One way of thinking about anxiety is that it is a reaction that happens when you can neither make sense out of events nor control them. It is common for many patients to feel anxious when they first go to the doctor: they cannot understand or make sense of what is wrong with them. When the doctor has explained what the problem is (even if their worst fears are confirmed), they often say they feel better. The same is true when we are waiting for the result of a test, or when we fear that a loved one no longer loves us. Even if the news is bad, at least we know. Indeed, most people say that the worst part is not knowing, and waiting.

So one of the best ways to help someone who is stressed and anxious is to give them information which will help to reduce their uncertainty: information reduces uncertainty. If uncertainty leads to anxiety, then it makes sense that telling someone about what is happening to them, and why, will reduce their uncertainty and anxiety. If patients do not know what to expect when they are asked to take some of their clothes off for an examination, or to go to the local hospital for 'tests', then they will try to guess what is likely to happen. Trying to make sense of things, they may remember films they have seen or stories they have heard, and perhaps frighten themselves totally unnecessarily. If patients knew what to expect they would not be so anxious. This does not mean that patients need to be flooded with technical terms. What it means is that when patients are involved and know about their treatment, they are much less likely to be anxious and stressed.

Research evidence shows that giving patients in hospital information about their hospital stay (like how long they are likely to remain in bed, what their operation entails, how much pain they will probably feel, and so on), actually reduces the length of their stay and cuts down on the amount of pain killers that they need. It has been found that if children who are in need of hospital care are told about hospitals and what to expect when they are admitted, then their recovery is quicker and easier. Ignorance is not bliss; it is an invitation to fear.

Cautionary notes

Two notes of caution need to be included here. Firstly, there seem to be some patients who really do not want to know what is wrong with them, and for whom providing information would be too frightening. For such people, information *increases* rather than decreases stress. However, this group is very much a minority, and they usually make it quite clear to their nurses and doctors that they do not wish to know. The nurse should of course respect that wish whilst bearing in mind the general rule, which is that patients want and benefit from more information.

The second cautionary note is that, when anxious, people are generally less able to concentrate, and find it harder to listen attentively to what is said to them. Therefore, it is sometimes necessary to repeat information again and again to get it through. Studies have shown that patients forget up to three-quarters of what is said to them in the doctor's surgery, *immediately after they have left the surgery*! These patients are not stupid, malicious, or trying to be uncooperative: the normal human being is simply not very good at remembering things when stressed. You should repeat information over and over again, or even write it down, so that all is clear in the patient's mind.

The stress of hospitalization

Having to be admitted to hospital for any reason can cause a lot of anxiety and stress.

1. New patients will be removed from everything that is familiar to them: their own home, their family, pets, and normal daily routines. Things which seem small and insignificant, like being able to have a cup of tea when you want one, a favourite television programme, or

even the sound of the children playing outside, are all important signals that you are secure and safe. Suddenly they are removed, and new sounds, sights and tastes are thrust upon the new and rather unwell patient. The stress of the unfamiliar is uncomfortable for everyone, but is especially likely to be disturbing for elderly patients and children, because they rely a lot on routine and familiarity.

2. As is normal in hospital, a number of unusual procedures are carried out which the patient frequently does not understand. Tests are carried out which are often left unexplained. Rather frightening equipment is used, which may appear very threatening. It may be necessary to use a bed pan, or remove clothes in front of strangers. Both these invasions of privacy and the new and strange happenings in the ward may be experienced as highly stressful.

3. The patient may be extremely worried about what is happening at home, especially if the admission was unexpected. The patient may be very worried by such questions as: Is someone looking after the children? Do the people at work know where to send my wages? Has anyone watered the tomatoes? These questions can sometimes seem more important than questions of life and death, and may prevent the person from relaxing and letting recovery take place.

4. Worst of all, patients often do not know what the future holds. The most pressing question is 'Will I get better?' Illness always implies the possibility of dying, and on that process, none of us has any information. It is of course very frightening not to know where you are going or how, which is what dying involves. For the relative or spouse of the dying person it can be equally or even more stressful, because they often do not know what to do to help. Bland reassurance does not really help very much. On the other hand, it does seem to be the case that understanding what is going on in the process of dying reduces the stress. Likewise, the relative of the dying person can be helped if information is given as to what is going on, what to expect, and what it is that the medical personnel are doing.

Being a patient in hospital is stressful and may well make recovery slower and more difficult. Much of the patient's energy is spent in coping with stress rather than regaining physical health. A community nurse who can help to relieve some of these anxieties before a patient goes into hospital may well significantly reduce the length of that patient's hospital stay, and increase the speed of recovery. In addition, a community nurse who can help both patients and relatives to understand the nature of the illness and treatment when at home will be able to prevent a lot of unnecessary suffering and anxiety. Just knowing that the community nurse will be there shortly after discharge from hospital is an additional way of reducing the stress and uncertainty of being in hospital.

WHAT CAN BE DONE TO REDUCE STRESS?

It has already been pointed out that what is stressful for one person is not necessarily stressful for another. In the same way, what helps one person to cope with stress will not necessarily do the same for everyone else. To an extent it is a question of trial and error, so that you have to decide what works for you or your patient on an individual basis. However, there are some well-known techniques of stress reduction and it is probably a good plan for community nurses who find themselves or their patients suffering from stress to try out some of these ideas as a way of reducing the pressures they feel.

Relaxation training

As we noted earlier, the physiological reactions to stress are automatic. If you sneak up behind someone and yell 'gottcha!', they will react according to the symptoms we noted. Thus it is almost impossible to separate the mental perception from the physical reaction. In other words, you cannot be mentally stressed and physically relaxed at the same time. The psychologist Edmund Jacobson noticed this connection and suggested that if people could be taught systematically to relax all of the muscles in their body then they would not simultaneously have feelings of tension and anxiety.

This is the basis of relaxation training: if we can interrupt or reverse each of the physiological reactions to stress, we can decrease the amount of stress felt. The process works like this:

1. Close your eyes. (Since we get approximately 75 per cent of our information input through our eyes, cutting down this stimulation is an important first step to relaxation.)

2. Start to breathe in regular, slow, deep breaths, but do not over-breathe, which can lead to feelings of dizziness. (Controlling breathing interrupts the rapid, shallow breathing that takes place during the stress reaction.)

3. Starting with either hand, make a fist as tight as you can without harming yourself. Notice where the tension lies. Then release the

fist and feel the tension flow out. Notice again how it feels now Feelings such as tingling or weightlessness are very common. No tice in particular the difference in feelings when the hand was tens and now that it is relaxed. Make a fist and relax it again and notice th difference once more.

4. Now do the same with the other fist. When you finish, notice th difference between your two hands and take just a moment and allov the least relaxed hand to become as relaxed as the other.

5. Follow the same process throughout all of the muscles in your whol body. Go from your hands through your arms, across your shoulder up your neck, down through your back, and into your legs, and finall your feet. Do not forget barely perceived groups of muscles such a your jaw and eye muscles.

6. Stop along the way to check if any of the muscle groups which yo have already relaxed have become re-tensed. If so, take a momen and allow them to re-relax. Remember that to make somethin, happen takes effort, which is the opposite to relaxation. In order t relax, you must *allow* it to happen. You cannot make it happen.

This fairly straightforward procedure has been found to be very helpf to people who are suffering from stress, as well as people who simpl want to be able to control how tense their body feels. It has also bee used for natural childbirth, where the relaxation training which is taugr to pregnant mothers is rather similar. Audio cassettes are widely avai able in which relaxation instructions can be played to the person wishin to learn how to relax, but there is no reason why individuals cannot do on their own. It needs a certain degree of determination to stick to it. T get the most benefit, relaxation has to be practised every day for abou 15 minutes or so, and it is a skill well worth acquiring.

People who do use relaxation exercises every day say it makes ther able to cope better with stressful situations when they occur suddenly as well as reducing their overall level of tension. Interestingly, som researchers have suggested that similar benefits can be obtained wit transcendental meditation, yoga and similar techniques. What they a have in common is that someone makes a decision to spend time quietl and peacefully, for a set period every day and acquire the skill c controlling bodily reactions instead of being controlled by them. It i certainly a cheaper and healthier method of relaxing than sedative alcohol or tranquillizers. If you do decide to recommend this form c self-help to patients, it would be sensible to try it out on yourself first.

Physical exercise

People who loved sport and physical education at school will be delighted to learn that it has now been established that physical exercise is good for your mental as well as physical health. Taking physical exercise is one of the best ways of coping with both stress and depression. A regular run or even a walk may be as effective as taking medication to deal with anxiety or depression. If you are feeling stressed, the chances are that you have started to neglect some of the physical activities that you used to enjoy, such as team games, swimming, cycling or dancing. All of these activities help, not only by getting the body moving and active, but also by getting people involved in something different and outside their own problems. Perhaps those gym teachers were right after all.

Sharing problems

The idea that sharing a problem halves it is well known. It does seem to be the case that people feel better once they have simply been able to talk over their difficulties with someone else. Getting the worries off your chest rather than bottling them up means you have to put into words things that you may not previously have thought through completely. The process of talking often puts things into perspective and allows you to think of new ways of seeing something that previously seemed to be permanent or insurmountable. Having a listener who is paying attention to you also tends to make you feel supported and valued. Thus it is that just talking about worries or preoccupations is a valuable stress-reduction technique.

This, of course, applies both to patients who are having to deal with the everyday stresses of life and to nurses who have to cope with all of their patients' problems. Turning first to the patient, everyone in the helping professions knows that sometimes the best thing to do for the patient or client is just to sit and listen, rather than to come up with particular solutions. What you are doing for other people when you sit and listen to them and their worries is to show them three important things:

- You are demonstrating that you care about them enough to give them time.
- You are showing them that you respect them enough not to think that your ideas are more important than theirs.

- You are making it clear that your aim is to help them sort out their own solutions to problems rather than impose your own solutions on them.

All of these three points are well known to good listeners. Indeed, the hallmark of a good listener is someone who keeps quiet for at least half of the time, asks lots of open questions, and does not make judgements.

This applies also to the support that friends or colleagues can give each other. If you feel stressed, find a friend who is willing to listen and share things with you. Again, you will probably know from experience of your own colleagues and friends that a good listener is one who gives you time and attention without imposing his or her own ideas or solutions on you. Alternatively, you can find a group of people in a similar situation who can provide a number of pairs of ears and constructive suggestions about how you could deal with things. More and more nurses have been setting up support and self-help groups. These exist in order to allow nurses to share their difficulties with one another. A valuable aspect of such groups is realizing that you are not alone, and that other people also feel the same way sometimes.

This applies to patients too, of course. Many self-help groups have been set up by patients or their relatives to provide support and sharing for group members. Self-help groups now exist for a vast range of conditions, from anorexia to Huntington's Chorea and from infertility to cancer. Such groups are undoubtedly very helpful to their members, and can help sufferers to talk about their problems in a supportive atmosphere, as well as providing useful hints and information about aids, grants available and money-raising ventures. But do not recommend a group unless you are sure that it is well led and responsibly run. A group that is poorly led or dominated by one or two individuals with a particular axe to grind may be less than helpful.

Medication

A very common response to someone who says they are feeling stressed, by both doctors and the general public, is to advise a prescribed course of tranquillizers, sedatives or sleeping pills. An enormous amount of medication is regularly prescribed for this reason. Millions of prescriptions for mood-altering drugs, such as Diazepam, are issued by doctors every year. People also medicate themselves with socially accepted drugs such as alcohol and tobacco, which also act as sedatives. They may in addition turn to increasingly popular illicit drugs, such as cocaine and marijuana.

Of course, there is nothing wrong with the use of either prescribed or legally available drugs to help someone over a particularly difficult crisis, but it is our view that the long-term use of drugs is likely to be unhelpful. This is because people are usually anxious and stressed *for some reason.* Just covering up the feelings of anxiety with pills is unlikely to take the problems away. As a short-term way of coping with unavoidable stress, such as an unexpected shock, sedatives are probably amongst the most 'painless' and common ways of coping. However, the tendency for people who are living in ways which make them unhappy (the unemployed, those in unhappy marriages, and so on) to rely for long periods of time on medication to make their lives bearable is regrettable. Anxiety and feelings of stress are not in themselves bad things: they are signals to the individual that something *is* the matter and needs to be changed. Alas, changing things is not always easy, which is probably why a prescribed solution to human problems seems so tempting.

CONCLUSION

In this chapter we have outlined the nature and causes of stress and suggested ways of coping with it. Given the hectic pace of modern life, and the pains and sorrows that beset us all at some time or other in our lives, it is not surprising that most people *do* feel stressed from time to time. Community nurses and health visitors, whose business it is to relate to people who are sick or in trouble, are more likely than most to encounter stressed people. It is therefore particularly important that they should have knowledge about stress as it is experienced by the families that they visit *and* as they themselves experience it. Perhaps it is a wounded healer who heals best in this area. If you sometimes feel under stress and can recognize and cope with it, this can give you an idea of how your patients must feel sometimes. However, it is also important to realize that people differ, in that what causes you to feel stressed may not have the same effect on someone else.

Because of the particular stresses experienced by nurses in carrying out their work, in the next chapter we discuss the results of prolonged stress on nurses. This has been called 'burnout', and is something which is increasingly causing concern to nurse managers and health administrators. We not only discuss what it is, but also what can be done about it.

Suggestions for further reading

Cox, T. (1978) *Stress*. London: Macmillan.
 One of the best all-round text books on the topic of stress, although it is fairly technical in parts. It will interest those who want a more academic approach.

Hayward, J. (1975) *Information: A prescription against pain*. London: Royal College of Nursing.
    Discusses the evidence for giving information to patients as a way of reducing stress.

Jacobson, E. (1978) *You Must Relax*. New York: McGraw.
Madders, J. (1980) *Stress and Relaxation*. London: Martin Dunitz.
Mitchell, L. (1977) *Simple Relaxation*. London: J. Murray.
Yendell, P. (1981) *Taking the Strain*. BBC Record: REC 407; BBC Tape: ZCM 407
    All of the above are sources of straightforward information about stress and some of the best ways of coping with it, such as relaxation and self-management. They can be used by nurses themselves as well as being suitable for patients.

Chapter 11

When the Batteries Go Flat: The Problem of Burnout

'I always know the danger signs,' said the nursing officer. 'It's when one of the nurses starts saying that she wished she worked in Marks and Spencers!' According to this nursing officer, colleagues who start talking about a desire to escape from nursing into a routine, less emotionally demanding job like being a shop assistant are on the road to disillusionment and despair about being a nurse. They are becoming 'burned-out' – the state both in hospital and the community when nurses start to lose energy, enthusiasm and commitment to a previously loved and fulfilling job.

Burnout, or the professional stress syndrome, is a serious threat to standards throughout the helping professions today. It results from a combination of factors which nursing, as well as other professions, has only recently started to recognize.

WHAT IS BURNOUT?

Burnout has been described as 'the sudden, depressed loss of interest in and capacity for work'. It affects all kinds of professional workers: teachers, chaplains, doctors and nurses. The signs are varied, and, of course, some may be symptoms of some other illness, or the expression of emotional problems which have nothing to do with work. Nevertheless, in the absence of a physical or mental illness or some emotional distress caused by family problems and the like, these signs may indicate the onset of burnout. Although so vague, and not as definite as an illness, it is useful to have a way of talking about something which is becoming more and more common in the nursing service. So we use the label, keeping in mind that it is not a disease or diagnosis, but simply a vivid way of talking about a not uncommon problem.

Among the various signs of burnout, not all will be seen in any one person, and they do not happen in any particular order. If you recognize some of these signs in yourself or your colleagues it does not mean you are all about to go down with some mysterious new affliction known as 'burnout', as you might go down with the flu. But it may mean that you are experiencing too much stress at work. This *does not* mean that you are at fault or personally to blame for feeling this way: quite the contrary. It means that you are having to work under continuously stressful conditions.

Nor does the fact that you may be feeling some of these things mean that you should give up your job right away. As with any disordered state, recognize the signs for what they are. This in itself helps, and allows you to start taking constructive action. Blaming yourself, or anyone else, is a singularly unhelpful thing to do, for it generally leads to recrimination and hopelessness. Self-blame is particularly unhelpful, as it rarely leads to constructive action. However, *you* are the only person that can do something about your future, and you are responsible for that. So if you do recognize these signs in yourself (assuming you are in good physical health), maybe it is worth thinking about what can be done to reduce your present level of stress at work by reducing your load to a point which is more manageable.

THE SIGNS OF BURNOUT

We can distinguish four different signs of burnout.

1. *Physical signs.*
A person may feel exhausted much of the time, will be susceptible to all sorts of minor illnesses like headaches, colds and coughs, and will need more and more days off work. Sleep may be disturbed. Smoking or alcohol intake may increase. A frequent problem is a loss of interest in sex, and a common preoccupation is weight – eating more and feeling increasingly depressed about a gain in weight. As a result, drastic and erratic diets are started, which, of course, do not work, leading to more feelings of depression. As burnout develops, nurses also say they never seem to have enough energy any more, so that even on days off there seems little point in going out or getting involved in things. Feelings of listlessness are common. In addition, the nurse may feel more and more tempted to rely on caffeine or self-medication to keep going. The big danger is of resorting to the inappropriate use of illegal or prescribed drugs as a way of coping. Not only will these not help in the long run, but, if discovered, can lead to dismissal or prosecution.

2. *Psychological signs.*

The nurse feels bored and sometimes unaccountably irritated with patients. At this point silly, rather insulting or degrading jokes will be made about patients, who are seen more as a nuisance than as the reason for doing the job. While jokes are sometimes used as a way of reducing tension, as in an operating theatre, the jokes which signal burnout are concealed expressions of contempt for patients. In this form, contempt is a desperate means for an individual to assert his or her own worth. These jokes are the sort which are not really funny, but are rather cruel and thoughtless.

In addition, the nurse may feel rather hopeless about the whole enterprise. A commonly heard cry is: 'What is the point of trying, when everything I try comes to no good in the end, anyway?' This despair then generalizes to others. Perhaps a new and idealistic member of staff joins the team, who makes some suggestions about possible improvements to the running of the ward or department, or has new skills and ideas to try out in the community. The common response by 'burned-out' staff to such suggestions is 'Oh no, that wouldn't work, we've tried that'. People who are idealists and have schemes or plans for improving the standard of care are seen at best as naïve fools, and at worst as troublemakers. Somehow, all of the ideas that inspired the nurse to enter nursing seem to have been shelved. What was a vocation becomes drudgery.

Another psychological sign is the nurse suddenly doing things out of character and on impulse and which may have destructive elements. Such impulses, like a dramatic resignation, may be a desperate attempt to regain control of an impossible situation. They may backfire, with unfortunate consequences. A resignation offered on impulse might be accepted!

3. *Social signs.*

These have to do with the relationships between people at home and at work. The number of conflicts increases. Arguments with colleagues and family will develop for no very good reason. Sometimes this can lead to the break-up of long-established relationships or even divorce. Becoming over-conscientious is another sign. There is always more to be done in the community, so there is enormous scope for overwork. Nurses may end up working 12 or 14 hours a day and still feel inadequate. This has a considerable impact on personal and family lives. Another nurse may go to the opposite extreme and do the absolute minimum. Patients are avoided at all costs, and the nurse feels oppressed and uncomfortable with both patients and colleagues.

4. *Institutional signs.*

These can be seen in the way that the hospital or community team works, rather than in one particular person. Low morale is a crucial factor, indicated by an increase in absenteeism and high staff turnover. There are of course many different reasons why people take time off sick or leave their jobs, but one of the reasons may simply be that they are fed up. Nursing managers are always worried about the high level of staff turnover, and a disturbingly large number of students leave as soon as they have qualified. This may indicate that all is not well with the job itself, and that students leave because they are aware of the dangers of impending burnout.

Another institutional sign is a growth in the number of disputes about who does what. The frequency and bitterness of demarcation disputes increase, so that more time is spent discussing who is responsible for a particular aspect of patient care than actually doing it. This comes from a tendency to focus on smaller and smaller things in an attempt to regain control, which gets worse when a high proportion of the staff are experiencing burnout. Related to this is the growth of sterile and frustrating staff meetings, which seem to get nowhere. Small groups of staff may also decide to boycott meetings.

Burnout spotters can also note the way in which staff will increasingly avoid patients and retreat into the office to do paperwork. Whilst the structure of the nursing profession does encourage this, in that promotion beyond the level of Sister or Charge Nurse almost inevitably involves losing regular contact with the patients, it can be observed in more junior staff, who will find all sorts of reasons to avoid interacting directly with patients. Managers for their part cease to be supportive of front-line care staff.

All of these signs point to less than happy (or efficient) staff. Patient care becomes a nuisance, and the nurse's own routine becomes more important than professional standards. Alternatively, the nurse may over-work until he or she drops from exhaustion. Yet at the same time the nurse recognizes that something is wrong, and that things just should not have turned out this way.

Burnout is best seen as an effort to cope with a high stress situation, and is actually an attempt by an individual to ensure their own psychological and physical survival, albeit at the cost of their idealism. We need, therefore, to understand why it comes about, and then to consider what we can do about it.

WHAT CAUSES BURNOUT?

In Chapter 10 we considered stress as an imbalance between the demands made of a person and their ability to meet those demands. Burnout, or professional work stress, is, therefore, best understood as what happens when the demands made by the job, as experienced by the professional, are greater than their own personal resources. So what is it about nursing which can be so stressful?

The emotional demand

The most important contributing factor to burnout in nurses is the *emotional* demand made by a job which involves unlimited caring for others who are in pain or in distress. Doctors, clergymen, social workers and teachers, too, have all detected burnout within their ranks. What all of these professionals share is the fact that they care for people on a day-to-day basis. This is a very personally demanding task. Although other aspects of being a nurse may be frustrating, it is the *emotional* aspect of the job which is particularly stressful, and which contributes most to burnout. It is, paradoxically, true that those nurses who are most involved in their jobs are the most likely to experience burnout.

We all accept that heavy physical work, such as shifting enormous weights like loads of bricks, furniture, coal or steel, is tiring, and we do not ask people to work like this without taking regular rest breaks. We do not ask people to do physical work without checking on safety, and if necessary providing lifting aids and training. Yet how do you measure the emotional 'work' involved in caring for a desperately ill child, or a distraught relative? Or how do you ensure that someone is taking enough emotional rest breaks? Or is it right to train nurses not to feel emotions, especially when we know that patients greatly appreciate and benefit from having a person nursing them who is emotionally responsive?

In the last chapter we noted that 'Interaction with significant people constitutes the most difficult sort of action required of us. People are decidedly the hardest thing we have to deal with.' The demands which caring for others places on our emotional strength can be just as exhausting as any physical task. Furthermore, there is no very simple way of restoring someone's emotional strength after a distressing encounter with a sick patient, in the way that there is of restoring someone's physical strength following completion of a strenuous physical task. If you are tired after a day of physical labour you can first sit down for a good meal, and then put your feet up. These two actions will restore your physical strength. But how do you restore someone's emotional strength? It is not at all clear.

If you are a caring person who automatically feels compassion for others, then just being with needy people is emotionally stressful. And some needy people cause more distress than others. Possibly the worst thing is having to deal with sick children, and feeling helpless and unable to do anything in the face of their pain, despite their trust in you. Or perhaps it is worse to deal with the dying, because of the finality of death. Some say that the worst thing is having to pretend that you are not affected by patients' distress, because that would be considered 'unprofessional' by other nurses. Whatever the cause of the emotional pain, nurses do not on the whole seem to have developed very good ways of helping each other to deal with distress.

Patsy was a very dedicated and efficient district nurse, who had to make regular visits to Eve, a middle-aged lady suffering from multiple sclerosis. Over the years of bathing and dressing Eve, Patsy had grown very fond of her patient, who was a cheerful and friendly person with tremendous courage and determination to make the best of her life despite her disabilities. To an extent, Patsy became part of the family, and was even invited to Eve's daughter's wedding. When Eve suddenly contracted pneumonia and died, Patsy was extremely upset, and asked to be allowed a day off duty to attend the funeral. Yet this request was refused, as Eve was considered not to have been 'family'. Indeed, when Patsy's senior found her crying at her desk the day after the death, Patsy was reprimanded for having 'got so involved'. She was told to 'pull herself together', and to show a 'good example' to the junior staff. This example of very real grief resulting from a bereavement, and managed in a punitive rather than supportive manner, might well lead to burnout.

There are a number of other possible causes of burnout in nurses. These we now examine briefly.

Lack of staff

It is a straightforward and perhaps unavoidable fact that many nurses work in a situation of chronic overload with inadequate staffing levels. Standards of care to which the nurse is trained have to be lowered or abandoned completely, with a resulting feeling of guilt and despair. The requirements of bureaucracy can be very frustrating, as more and more time gets swallowed up doing paperwork or going to meetings. The nurse who wants to spend time with patients may have to spend endless hours on the telephone, or writing letters, which all take time away from the patients. Being so busy means that when there *is* time to spend with a patient, the nurse is always surreptitiously watching the clock, and spending at least half the time calculating how to get the next three appointments fitted in before the end of the day.

Lack of training

The next source of stress which can lead to burnout is the unfortunate fact that many nurses simply do not feel that they have had suitable training to do the job that they are supposed to be doing. This inevitably creates a lack of confidence and a feeling that they are doing things 'on the run', as well as a sense that they are letting down their patients.

Joanna, a district nurse, was asked to take over the care of Bobby, a severely mentally handicapped boy who was being transferred from the local hospital to live with his parents in the community. Although Joanna had received a basic introduction in the care of the mentally handicapped when doing her community training, she felt almost totally inadequate when faced by the boy's parents, desperate for help when Bobby suddenly started head banging. Joanna remembered something about the need to establish programmes to cope with such behaviour, but she really didn't know where to start. She visited the family a few times to attempt to deal with the problem, but in the end had to give up in despair when everything she tried seemed to fail. She felt she had just made things worse by interfering.

Often nurses do not feel able to ask for help, because they feel they *ought* to know, despite being aware that their training has been inadequate. They also know that the amount of specialist time available is never adequate, and so feel obliged to try to help their patients even though they know their attempts are likely to be unsuccessful. This kind of situation is a ripe source of the stress which leads to burnout.

Lack of recognition

Connected with the experience of inadequacy is the opposite feeling: that of *not* being recognized or valued for what you *can* do. Sadly it is still the case that some doctors do not treat nurses very well and see them as 'handmaidens' who are there to act as personal servants rather than as colleagues. It is demoralizing to feel that one's own work is being undervalued, and someone else is getting all of the recognition, especially when a special effort has been made with a particular patient. Lack of recognition can lead to feelings of being unwanted, unappreciated and bitter. Most of us are not in a job where our patients reward us directly, so the sense of doing a good job is especially important. Feedback from our seniors lets us know we are doing a good job. Getting no praise at all is very depressing, especially when working in the more difficult or chronic areas of nursing, where even the satisfaction of patients getting better is often missing.

Lack of communication

Working with seriously ill patients, when communication within the team is not very well organized, can also be very stressful. Patients often feel easier when talking to nurses than doctors about tricky subjects, and will often ask nurses the questions about diagnosis and prognosis which they have not dared to ask their doctor. If the nurse does not know what the patient has been told, or is working with a doctor who believes that patients do not need to know, it can make life very difficult. Equally frustrating is when the nurse's own advice on the subject is disregarded by the doctor, apparently for no very good reason. Responses of frustration and helplessness are hardly surprising in such circumstances.

Working with the terminally ill

Another cause of burnout is, of course, the regular encounter that many nurses have with death. We discussed this at length in Chapter 5, so will not repeat the discussion here, except to say that for some particularly caring nurses, the stress may not be apparent for many years. Just as soldiers in battle sometimes do not seem to feel the stress until months or even years after the war is over, so too nurses may not immediately show the results of the pressures that they have been living under for some time. This delayed reaction is known as 'post-traumatic stress reaction', and is often seen with nurses who have to deal very closely with intense situations such as death and do not have the opportunity to cope with the stress properly at the time. A number of different reactions can be seen, such as vivid dreams or 'flash-backs', or else difficulties in getting emotionally close to anyone at all.

The stress of trying to be Superman or Superwoman!

A further cause of burnout is more personal, and has to do with the fact that the types of demands being made in the daily routine of nursing may in fact be rather similar to those being made in the home. It is still the case that most nurses are women, which means that nurses share with other working women the problems of having to do two jobs: the professional, paid job of nursing, and the unpaid job of housework. Whilst many husbands and boyfriends agree to the idea of helping with the housework and sharing child-care, this is often only lip-service. The responsibilities of the home still tend to get left to the woman. A recent survey reported that working women spend up to five times as much time doing housework as their husbands! This means that, for some nurses at least, they have to go home, after spending the whole day cleaning up after and dispensing care and advice to distressed patients, to spend the evening cleaning up after and giving care and advice to demanding children – not to mention a demanding husband too!

Even more tiring than the business of having to come home and do housework on top of a difficult job is the fact that nurses on the whole tend to be better at giving attention and emotional care to people than taking it. All too often they struggle on without asking for help themselves. Added to this, many working mothers are likely to feel some anxiety or guilt about their decision to work and will therefore be less likely to ask for help even if they need it.

A health visitor with ten years' experience, Carol had three young children. Gary, who worked in the computer industry, was a sympathetic but rather ambitious husband. One of the children, Amanda, had a severe speech impediment. When Carol and Gary married and decided to have children they agreed that Carol should return to work when the children were old enough, and that they would as far as possible share the child-care. Their relationship was a good one, and Carol found that Gary was always willing to listen and encourage her when she had a particularly difficult case to deal with at work.

However, a few months after Carol had gone back to work full-time, Gary was offered an excellent position in a very dynamic company. Although the job did not pay very well, the prospects seemed good. Unfortunately, the job meant that Gary had to spend quite a few evenings working each week. Consequently he no longer had time to talk things over with Carol as they used to. In addition, Carol resolved that she must not burden Gary with too many domestic or work problems at this point in his career. Although she knew that she and Gary had originally agreed to share child-care and housework, she felt somehow that her career was not as important as Gary's, so that she should take the lion's share in arranging care for the children. She also felt that since she was in full-time employment, unlike many of the wives of Gary's new colleagues, she must take special care in maintaining high standards of entertaining and housework, 'not to let the side down'.

Gradually Carol developed an almost impossible schedule for herself: she would be up at around six o'clock in the morning to do the housework before packing sandwiches for all the family. Then she would take the children to their schools or childminders before arriving at work. She spent most lunch hours doing the family shopping or errands. Evenings were spent helping the children with their homework, entertaining Gary's colleagues, or listening to Gary's worries about his new responsibilities. She also managed to fit in Amanda's visits to the speech therapist. Although she knew she was getting more and more exhausted, Carol could not seem to blow the whistle, feeling somehow that she 'ought' to do all of this, as a good wife and mother.

In addition, things at work were getting more difficult, for Carol was herself being asked to take on additional responsibility. She was respected in the practice in which she worked, being seen as a competent and caring person who could be trusted with some of the most difficult cases. Despite being tired, Carol never missed or was late for appointments, and seemed to show considerable sensitivity and judgement when dealing with a couple of cases of non-accidental injury. As the mother of a handicapped child herself, Carol knew how important it is to give plenty of time and attention to parents who are having difficulties with their children, and was therefore prepared to invest a lot of energy in helping these particular families. But what no one realized was that from time to time Carol would find herself bursting into tears as she drove around between visits, and once or twice she had to stop the car in a deserted car park until she managed to stop crying. She was drinking more and more coffee, just to keep going. Because she felt she was not working as well as she used to, and was anxious about being seen as unable to cope with her new responsibilities by her seniors, she volunteered to take over responsibility for the students attached to the practice. In order to keep up with her additional paperwork, she spent the evenings working after the children had gone to bed.

Then catastrophe threatened. Gary's new firm was suddenly on the verge of collapse, and one of the new doctors in Carol's practice turned out to be a real slave-driver who was always critical of Carol's best efforts. On one occasion, the new doctor insisted that Carol miss a number of visits and rewrite all of her case records, because he didn't like the way she had been doing them in the past. Carol wondered what on earth she was bothering for, and almost imperceptibly began to give up the effort. She found that she was quite easily able to pass new patients on to the students, and if she was careful could spend quite a few afternoons each week on 'administration'. She also reasoned that there was no point worrying about being punctual for appointments. Since there were so many patients in need, what did her contribution matter anyway? She decided that she had been very foolish in the past for bothering so much about the families that she had to visit, and that she would simply do the minimum required. She did notice that somehow she hadn't been getting so much satisfaction from her job lately, and also that her relationship with Gary wasn't so good any more. But she was so tired. Gradually she came to accept that she was not the excellent, caring nurse that she had always wanted to be. She was in fact no different from all those old battle-axes that she used to despise when she was training herself. But after all, she now understood that it was all hopeless anyway, and her efforts were not going to make any impact on the unmet needs that she saw around her. So why bother?

It is not productive to try and find someone to 'blame' for Carol's distress. She was simply exhausted, and unable to find any more emotional or physical strength to cope. Believing that she should be an unending source of strength to others, she had no appreciation of her own limitations. So in the end she simply gave up. Perhaps she should have confided in one of her seniors. Yet it is surprising how infrequently nurses do feel able to take problems to senior staff, who are perhaps in a position to do something about stress levels. Perhaps she should have confided in Gary, her husband. In fact, one of the most helpful things a person can do if they are stressed is to talk to spouse or friends. This does not mean that the spouse or friend has to come up with the answers. In fact, the spouse who comes up with 'solutions' is often not seen as being as helpful as the spouse or partner who simply listens and sympathizes. But in any case, Gary was too busy worrying about himself. Or maybe he was just seen by Carol as being too busy.

Perhaps what Carol could have done was to recognize the signs of burnout in herself – spells of crying, an attempt to work harder and harder, reliance on caffeine and so on. The attempt to become 'Supernurse' may be encouraged by the journals we read and television programmes we watch, but is bound to result in failure and guilt sooner or later.

WHAT CAN WE DO ABOUT BURNOUT?

Burnout results from a dilemma. Patients value and benefit from emotional and personal contact with nurses who are prepared to give of themselves. Yet this giving leads to exhaustion in the nurse. So what can we do about it?

Nurses working in emotionally demanding jobs on the verge of burnout have one of three options open to them.

- They can simply do their best and then resign or change jobs. It may be that the high turnover in nursing actually represents the attempt by some nurses to cope with their stresses, and should not be seen as a bad thing. But of course it is not an ideal solution for the nursing profession, because many gifted and sensitive nurses leave before they are really able to make much of a contribution. Nor is it an ideal solution for the individual, who must have invested a considerable amount of energy and commitment in training in the first place.

- Nurses can simply set limits to what they expect of themselves, and refuse to do more than is reasonable. This may involve changes within the structure of nursing teams so that no one individual is asked to take on too many cases without support. But it may also mean that changes have to occur within people's personal lives, so that we do not expect professionals to take on too many emotionally demanding tasks at once. Too many nurses under stress are almost certainly trying to do everything: being resourceful parents who are always there to help their children; supportive partners who always have time for their spouse's worries; excellent hosts or hostesses; inspiring teachers or supervisors; dynamic team leaders; outstanding professionals who really care for their patients; and so on. But it just cannot be done by mere mortals, which, after all, is what we all are.

- Maybe nurses at all levels of nurse management have to spend some time working out effective ways of coping with stress within the profession. In other words, perhaps the profession as a whole has to start to recognize the problem of burnout and attempt to do something about it.

Before discussing these ways of coping, a general point must be made. If you do have the opportunity of trying out some of these ideas remember that no one should be forced to take part in a 'burnout eliminating plan' against their will. Not everyone will find your idea of reducing burnout is the right one for them.

STRATEGIES FOR DEALING WITH BURNOUT

1. Nurse counsellors

Some nursing departments, particularly in large hospitals, have arranged for a trained counsellor to be available for nurses working in particularly stressful areas, so that nurses can have someone to talk to about the problems that arise in the work place. This person may be a nurse or another professional, such as a chaplain or psychologist. Nurses who feel stressed are therefore able to go to see someone in complete confidence to discuss situations that have been particularly upsetting. As a result of the advice and support which is given by the counsellor, levels of stress are never allowed to build up to the point where burnout is the only possible result. It is important that this counsellor should not be a part of the formal nursing hierarchy, so that anything that is said in a counselling session is not used against that nurse at a later date, for example when promotion is being considered. This might be an idea for community nursing departments to consider too, as stress levels can be higher in the community than in hospitals, and burnout is as much a risk in the one setting as the other.

2. Support groups

The idea of support groups has already been mentioned in Chapter 10. Simply knowing that other people are feeling the same way, and have the time and concern to listen to you when you have had a particularly hard day, can in itself be helpful. Groups like this can help to check up on how much work people are doing: *not* to see if they are doing enough, but rather to make sure they are not doing too much, and thus endangering their survival as nurses in the longrun. Another role for these groups is simply to make sure that nurses are taking enough time for themselves, and 'recharging their batteries'.

Of course support groups are not the only way of recharging batteries. It is possible to be supportive to other nurses by just making sure that you do provide time for a distressed colleague to talk or cry after a particularly difficult or emotionally demanding visit. It is also possible to be supportive by persuading colleagues to try to take on only a manageable workload. The effect of giving time and attention to someone who feels drained is to allow them a chance to recharge their batteries. No one can go on giving unless they sometimes get resourced themselves.

3. Stress management training

Many nurses feel somewhat aggrieved that no one ever really prepared them during training for the stresses to come when they eventually qualified. They complain that the time they spent in school did not properly deal with the real problems they were to face in the world outside. Certainly, very few schools run courses on stress management, or put on sessions concerned with personal survival. But, particularly in the United States, some schools of nursing are now providing courses on anxiety-management skills, as well as relaxation classes. Both these strategies help. Just knowing what to expect often allows people to cope much better. There seems to be no reason why such sessions should not be held in Great Britain or elsewhere. We all know that prevention is better than cure. Perhaps the nursing profession should recognize this within its own ranks, and do something constructive about it during nurse training.

4. Flexible shift and holiday patterns

Sometimes, despite all our best intentions, and despite supportive friends, colleagues and family, it all becomes too much. We simply need a break. It is important that nurses are able to have not only regular breaks from work, but also the occasional 'irregular' break, when the pressure is too great. This break should not have to be taken as sick leave but should be available when someone has been under too much pressure for too long. Even an afternoon off may be enough in some cases. What is done with that time off will vary. Not all people find support from talking over their worries with friends or colleagues, but instead they may find it most relaxing to spend time on their own, doing physical exercise, or doing domestic things like baking bread or cooking. Whatever they choose to do, it is important to realize that this time is not 'wasted' from the point of view of nursing management. On the contrary, it may well help to prevent the nurse from becoming burned out, or leaving nursing completely. It is in fact another way of replenishing resources.

5. Improved communications and feedback

A major source of stress in nursing, as in many other working situations, arises when there is poor communication within teams, wards or units. Two different types of communication breakdown are most closely linked to burnout.

- The first happens when senior staff are too busy or too uninterested to bother to let junior staff know what is happening, or to ask for their opinion. Not knowing what the plans of the team or ward are can lead to feelings of frustration and helplessness that can in turn lead to burnout. Too many nurse managers seem to forget what it was like when they were junior nurses, and do not make the time to explain things, or to ask for ideas and opinions. As a result, not being consulted creates the sense of being undervalued and not having any real contribution to make. Of course, the nurse managers may themselves be working under pressure and feeling the same way about *their* managers in turn . . . But the result is bad feelings all round, and an experience of not being valued or even taken into consideration.

- The second form of communication breakdown takes place when senior nurses or nurse managers fail to give appropriate feedback to junior nurses about their work. As we have already pointed out, patients are not really in a position to recognize and appreciate some of the difficulties and problems of being a nurse, and whilst some patients and relatives can be very grateful for their nursing care, others can be very ungrateful and even violent or aggressive. It is crucial therefore that someone *does* recognize the worth of the effort that has been made. Staff appraisal forms are one way of doing this, although they are not popular with everyone.

It may be that the best way of making sure that you get encouragement is in fact to train your boss to give it to you! This involves making it clear to your manager or senior colleague that you would like regular feedback from him or her, and pointing out how valuable you find the feedback you are given. You may be pleasantly surprised by what you hear, and it may help you to realize how much your work is appreciated. Or you may hear realistic criticism which does at least feel like real feedback and give you something to work on. The important thing is that everyone needs to be valued and to get feedback, no matter how long they have been in the job.

IN CONCLUSION

We have devoted a whole chapter to the subject of staff burnout because we feel it is a major issue in all of the caring professions, including nursing. Yet many nurses fail to notice burnout within their ranks, let alone within themselves. Not noticing it is not going to make it go away, however. The first step to dealing with the problem, as with other problems, is to recognize its existence and extent. Only then can you start to think of ways of dealing with it. An emotionally-drained nurse is not going to be a good nurse, or even one who stays around for very long. There are no easy solutions, but we hope that in this chapter we have presented a few ideas. Nurses cannot go on giving for ever, as their resources will be exhausted. And that will not benefit anyone, least of all the patients.

Suggestions for further reading

Jacobson, S. and McGrath, H. (1983) *Nurses under Stress*. Chichester: Wiley.
Provides an account of the stresses experienced by nurses in a variety of specialized settings.

Llewelyn, S.P. (1984) The cost of giving: Emotional growth and emotional stress. In: S. Skevington (ed.) *Understanding Nurses: The social psychology of nursing*. Chichester: Wiley.
This chapter discusses some of the feelings likely to be experienced by both patients and nurses. It shows how responding as a person to patients' pain or distress can be extremely hard on nurses. The need for adequate support is emphasized and suggestions are made for ways of providing such support.

Maslach, C. (1981) *Burnout: The cost of caring*. Englewood Cliffs, N.J.: Prentice Hall.
Written by one of the best-known authors in the field of burnout, this book provides a detailed account of work-induced stress, its causes, symptoms and consequences. It covers a wide variety of professional groups, including nurses.

Chapter 12

The Professional Nurse: Working Together and Alone

In this last chapter, we look at the profession of nursing in the community, where nurses within a team nevertheless shoulder a great deal of individual professional responsibility and isolation. Herein lie many of the tricky parts of the job.

- Firstly, we look at some of the areas of conflict and cooperation often experienced when people work in groups or teams.
- Secondly, we look at some of the problems involved in working alone and consider how best nurses can develop their professional skills when handling difficult situations on their own.
- Finally, we look briefly at the overall importance of nursing in the community.

WORKING IN GROUPS

'I love nursing, it's a great gob. The part I like best is being with the patients. But the part I can't stand is all the wrangling between nurses, or between the Community Nursing Service and Social Services, or between the day nurses and the night nurses. Why do people have to spend so much time arguing with each other, when we all know it is the patients that matter?'

Most of us in health care could echo the anguished question asked by this nurse. Anyone who works in a complex organization knows that lots of time and energy is spent arguing with other people about apparently silly things, like who is going to foot the bill for some particular service when it all comes out of the public purse, anyway; or who is going to be

161

responsible for organizing some aspect of patients' treatment when we are all aiming for the same goal after all.

Often the people with whom we spend most of our time arguing are the people whose work is most similar to our own. In hospitals, rivalries seem to develop between groups of staff on the same ward, for example between enrolled and registered nurses, or between nurses and occupational therapists. Sometimes the rivalries may spring up between the day nursing staff and the night duty staff on the same ward, or else between trained staff and students. Occasionally this conflict between groups can become so bitter that patient care does start to suffer, because members of the two groups in conflict stop communicating with each other as mutual trust and respect breaks down. Why does this happen, and what can be done about it?

Groups and identity

Conflict is bound up with our sense of our own identity. In order to understand why this is the case, we need to look at the process by which a sense of identity is developed.

As this book is about nurses, let us use nurses as an example. Whether you are an enrolled nurse, a health visitor, a psychiatric nurse, a midwife, a school nurse or a member of the teaching staff, the exact group to which you belong is likely to be very important to you. Possibly you believe, deep down, that *your* type of nursing is the most interesting, or the most important, or the most caring of all of the branches of nursing. In other words, you feel some special loyalty towards and pride in your particular group.

People do not become nurses overnight. It requires commitment, dedication and a great deal of hard work and painful experience before the satisfaction of professional certainty and the regard of patients begins to develop. Being a nurse eventually becomes a very important part of someone's life, crucial to self-regard and a sense of personal value. A large part of who we are is defined by what groups we belong to.

We also have to learn what to do in order to belong to a particular group, and hence to gain this valuable boost to our sense of identity. One of the ways you learn to be a part of the group is by behaving like other group members. For example, on most hospital wards new learners are encouraged to watch trained nursing staff, and to model themselves on the trained nurses. They are encouraged to imitate those who are already group members, and behave as they do. In this way, new learners are taught to identify themselves as professional nurses. In this way our sense of identity (who we are) is heavily dependent on what groups we choose to belong to (who we choose to be like), which in turn is defined by what we do.

This can be demonstrated as follows. Count up all of the groups (or groupings) to which you belong and you will probably find they number almost three dozen. For example, you may be a member of the female part of the human race; in addition you may be British; a nurse; a member of the Smith family; a Roman Catholic; you may belong to the Frank Sinatra fan club (even if you do not often admit to it); you may be an occasional member of your local darts team. There is probably no one else in the world who belongs to exactly the same combination of groups as you do. If you continue counting for long enough you will find that by describing your different group memberships you will have described all the particular parts of your life and that if anyone was listening they would have a pretty good idea of what you thought was interesting, important and entertaining. In other words, your listener could make a reasonably shrewd guess about the kind of person you are even if they could not say for sure whether you were a nice or a nasty person.

So in many ways knowing what groups someone belongs to tells us who they are. Of course it does not tell us in detail what kind of person they are, but it does tell us quite a bit about their interests and what opinions they are likely to hold about a whole range of topics.

All of this has two consequences. The first is that our group membership is actually very important to us in giving us identity. The second is that we all continually make judgements about other people based on *their* group membership. These judgements may or may not be accurate. We illustrate these two points in turn.

- Firstly, the crucial importance of group membership to a person's sense of identity can be demonstrated by looking at people who have lost their jobs. Besides the economic consequences of being unemployed, jobless people often say they feel that they have lost their sense of 'being someone', and will report a sense of being a non-person, or even as being 'on the scrap-heap'. In other words, they have lost some of their sense of identity. Sometimes housewives say the same thing, since having a job is a very strong source of identification.

- Secondly, the way in which we make judgements about other people on the grounds of their group membership can be demonstrated by looking at the way that we make assumptions about other nationalities. For example, we may say that all Italian people are fat and lazy; or all Americans are loud-mouthed and brash. This process, known as stereotyping, leads us to lump people together as a group, and to make broad sweeping statements about them, often without any evidence or proof. Stereotyping can be a process akin to stigmatizing.

Group comparison and conflict

These two points help us to understand why there is often so much conflict between groups of staff in health care settings like hospital teams, or general practices. A natural way of simultaneously finding out who you are and finding out who someone else is to compare yourself with the other person. This often means comparing *your* group with *their* group. It takes a very unusual person to be able to compare the group they belong to with another group that they do not belong to and *not* to think their group is better (although this does not exclude envying others for some of their qualities or possessions). Most people naturally think that their group, whether it is their family, their football team, their hospital, their school or their nation, is the best. Even if their group may not be as successful, or as rich or as big as another group, nevertheless it may well seem better in some other way: it is friendlier, or more in touch with reality or more hard-working. After all, how many supporters of Manchester United football club actually think that Liverpool is a better team? And how many Americans actually think that Great Britain is a better place to live? And vice versa? In fact, if they did so they might be called disloyal, or even labelled a traitor. So belonging to a group almost inevitably means comparing your group with other groups and, very frequently, reaching the conclusion that your group is better. Of course, this reflects well on you and boosts your pride in your own identity. After all, who would want to belong to a group which was worse than the other groups around? Groucho Marx's famous comment, that he would not want to join a club which wanted him as a member, was based on his belief that any club which admitted him *must* be no good!

This process of comparison and loyalty to one's own group lies at the root of lots of positive emotions, like patriotism, team loyalty and family pride. So long as groups are not in conflict about anything serious these loyalties are beneficial and make people proud to be who they are. The problems start when healthy competition between groups develops into aggressive rivalry or even open warfare. Then we start finding out or even inventing all sorts of negative things about the other group, such as the idea that they are evil, unclean, lacking in intelligence or self-seeking. This simultaneously makes us feel even prouder to be who we are (even if our confidence needs artificial boosting) and even more sure of our fragile superiority to the others. And of course they may be saying precisely the same things about us.

The development of rivalries usually happens under two conditions.

- Firstly, when there is a shortage of resources, so that there is no longer as much to go around as there used to be. When that happens, people start to defend their own groups and dismiss the claims of other groups to have a share.
- Secondly, when people do not see much of each other, and do not have the chance to learn the truth about the other group: that they too are human, and have lots of positive qualities as well. Consequently, it is possible to build up all sorts of prejudices and stereotypes about the others and never find out whether they are true or not.

It will perhaps have become obvious by now that this process of competition and stereotyping is what goes on whenever there are wars, or where there is colour prejudice or religious bigotry. In simple terms both sides think that they are right and good, and that the other side is evil and wicked. In addition, each side feels extremely proud to belong to *their* group, which gives them a strong sense of identity, and also makes them even more determined not to give in to the other side.

Group conflict in the health services

But it does not take national conflict to mobilize these resources. It is extremely instructive to look closely at what is happening when there is conflict between groups in our workplaces. Obviously, conflict is not as serious in most hospitals or health teams as it is in wartime or between rival football teams: all groups working in the health services *do* want the same thing – the welfare of the patient. Nevertheless, we know that some typical negative aspects of conflict do happen between groups of nurses, such as stereotyping, or always blaming the others when things go wrong. An awful lot of time is wasted in moaning about 'the others', who never seem to be as hardworking or caring as we are. It can sometimes be even more serious than this, when *they* (it is almost always them, not us) stop communicating with *us*. When one group, say nurses in Hospital A, start to believe that they are the only ones who really know how to look after patients, and that the nurses in Hospital B are incompetent or inferior, then it is only a matter of time before patient care starts to suffer as communication breaks down between Hospital A and Hospital B.

Reducing group conflict

The solutions which can be applied to conflicts between groups of nurses are in fact the same as those which can be applied to nations at war, or to groups of religious zealots who are in conflict with each other. Unfortunately, it is very much easier to set up and prolong conflict between groups than it is to break down conflict and promote peace. But it is important to try.

1. Education.

The first thing to do when trying to reduce conflict between groups is to help people to have some sort of understanding about what is happening. Just realizing that 'they' see you in exactly the same way as you see 'them' can sometimes put things in perspective. It can make you realize how unproductive it is to spend all of this time and energy blaming other people, when they are doing just the same to you. Understanding why conflicts grow up between groups may start the process of reconciliation. Education is clearly important here in helping people to see what they are doing, and why.

2. Communication.

The second and possibly the most important way to reduce conflict between groups is communication. If we do not have regular contact with other people we can develop all sorts of derogatory ideas about them which may not in fact be true. Then we make judgements about them which are merely based on prejudice and bias. However, if we communicate with people the chances are that we will discover that they are not as unlike us as we thought. They have feelings and fears just like us, and may be as interested as we are in developing a better relationship.

Pam was a district nurse working in a very busy and rather run-down inner-city practice, who had little time or inclination for chatting to nurses in other areas. In particular, she felt rather irritated by some of the nurses who worked in a neighbouring area which had a mainly middle-class population. She felt that they didn't really know anything about the very difficult urban problems that she had to face, and that they probably spent most of their time drinking tea with their patients.

*When one of Pam's particularly difficult patients was transferred to
an estate across the city she was asked to hand over care for this patient
to Marta, a nurse from the 'nice' middle-class practice, and to explain to
Marta some of the particular problems of the case. Pam was very
scathing about this, feeling she had better things to do than waste her
time talking to Marta. Consequently, she didn't bother to return a
series of telephone calls which Marta made enquiring about the patient.
On the one occasion when Pam did try to call back, Marta was out on
a visit, and Pam's immediate thought was 'Oh, yes. I bet she's just
knocked off work early. Typical of these middle-class nurses, who haven't
a clue about the real world!' So she didn't even bother to leave a
message. In the meantime, Marta was struggling with a series of very
tricky cases in her 'nice' middle-class area, and grew increasingly
irritated with Pam, who worked in that inefficient and dirty inner-city
practice. So Marta soon abandoned all attempts to contact Pam, who
probably spent most of her time with her feet up, drinking tea with her
patients . . .*

*It so happened that a few weeks later, Pam was attending a one-day
course for nurses working with patients in the community who were
suffering from terminal cancer. Part of the course involved small group
discussions about the problems and difficulties involved in supporting and
encouraging such patients. Pam was struck by some of the sensitive and
helpful comments being made by one of the other nurses on the course,
who spent some time describing the particular stresses of her own job. To
Pam's immense surprise, she discovered that this helpful and perceptive
nurse turned out to be none other than Marta. This unexpected
meeting allowed the two nurses to share their experiences and, in time,
to laugh about the way each had developed a negative and stereotyped
view of the other. These views had been based on their prejudiced
opinions of nurses who belonged to a different group from their own.
Through better communication each nurse learned how wrong their
prejudiced view of the other group had been.*

What Pam and Marta had at first failed to do was to communicate with
each other, so that they could both learn something about each other's
difficulties. Both of them developed stereotypes about the other, and this
made things much worse. The person who might have suffered was the
patient who had been transferred across the city.

If we do not make the effort to communicate we almost always start
misunderstanding the other person or group, and this leads very easily to
a position where we resolve *not* to communicate with them anyway. So

the cycle of misunderstanding, stereotyping and rivalry goes on, and gets more and more serious, unless something happens to disrupt the cycle.

3. Changing places.

The third way to break down some of the rivalries and antagonisms that tend to build up between groups is to encourage people to swap places from time to time. This is why it is such a good idea for nurse tutors to spend time on the ward, and for trained staff to spend time in school. Another useful move is for more senior staff to spend time working with their more junior colleagues, on the ward or in the community. This has two benefits. It allows more junior staff to see that people further up the nursing hierarchy are human too, and it prevents the senior or administrative staff from forgetting what it is like to be actively involved with patients. On the other hand, it is also useful for junior staff to go along to some of the apparently endless and unproductive meetings which often take up the time of nurses involved in management so that they can see what is involved. Without this kind of exchange it is very easy for stereotypes to develop: for example the idea that junior nurses are irresponsible and are not dedicated to their jobs; or, on the other hand, the idea that senior staff are simply having a good time and do not care in the slightest about their juniors.

Decisions, decisions . . .

Sometimes teams spend an awful lot of time reaching decisions, or, rather, failing to reach decisions. Unless there is a skilled person running or chairing a meeting it is possible to waste the time and enthusiasm of a large number of people. Meetings which are weakly chaired can degenerate into boring wranglings about trivial subjects between people who do not seem to be listening to each other anyway, while really important issues get left to the end or even delayed to the next meeting. But another danger can arise when the person who is running the team takes *too* much control and does not allow other members of the team enough time to express their own ideas. We all know leaders of teams who seem to only be interested in voicing their own opinions. Someone like this is not likely to be a very good team leader, and will soon lose the cooperation and enthusiasm of the other team members.

In addition, meetings are expensive, they can involve a lot of people, and time is money. Sometimes teams or meetings are asked to make decisions, or to complete tasks, which are in fact best made by individuals, as, for example, how to compose a letter of thanks or complaint. On these occasions, most of the people at the meeting have nothing to do, and just have to sit there feeling bored and frustrated. It would be far better to delegate such tasks to an individual or pair of individuals, rather than use up the valuable time of the whole committee membership.

Teamwork and leadership

Although we have concentrated here on some of the unhelpful aspects of working in groups, it is true that groups do have many benefits. These include being able to offer support and advice to group members, as well as often being the most efficient way of getting a job done. Most of us work in teams because it would be physically impossible for us to do all of the jobs that need to be done on our own. Many general practices now employ a wide assortment of staff, including doctors, nurses, counsellors, receptionists and secretaries, because they recognize that there is too much work for any individual doctor or nurse to do alone. In addition, having a large number of staff in the practice or team means that people can specialize and develop particular skills. This saves time all round. Teams and groups are effective if care is taken in their management and leadership.

It is perhaps obvious that being a good leader involves real skill. It requires the ability to make decisions, and, perhaps even more important than this, to be good listener. You cannot make decisions if you do not listen to what your team has to say. One way of learning team leadership skills is to watch good leaders very carefully, and see how it is that they do it. You will probably notice that they avoid having too many meetings, but that when they do they make sure that everybody has a say, including the quietest and most unimportant member of the team. For there is no connection between how much people talk and how many sensible things they have to say. A good leader will make sure that the loud and dominant personality in a team does not completely overwhelm the quieter and more thoughtful person. A good leader will also make everyone feel that their contribution is welcomed, no matter how small. But being organized is important, too. Simply paying attention to obvious things like having an agenda, sticking closely to time limits, setting objectives for the meeting, and so on, means that the team can make decisions effectively.

Teams or groups are important in helping people to achieve a sense of identity. But this does not only result in negative things like prejudice and conflict. It also results in pride, professional standards and a strong sense of professional commitment. These are obviously good and positive aspects of belonging to groups, which may help to explain why most of us still value groups and teamwork, despite the snags.

WORKING ON YOUR OWN

Nurses in the community regularly have to take an enormous amount of responsibility for their patients without the back-up of a team right behind them. Even if the team will help in the longrun, when you are out on your own the support can seem an awfully long way away.

There are two situations in which working on your own can be a special problem:

- when you are taken advantage of or abused, verbally, physically or sexually
- when you are asked to make decisions or give advice which you know is outside your sphere of competence.

Both experiences can be very unnerving, especially if you have not anticipated them. But even if you know that these things sometimes happen they can still make you feel tremendously anxious. We look at each of these problems in turn.

Dealing with the violent patient

Patients respond in a violent way when they are either frightened or frustrated. Most of us have learned, when we do not get what we want, to put up with the situation and to wait until another time. But some patients are not very good at tolerating frustration and may use violence or abuse to try and get their way. Alternatively, patients may become aggressive when they are in pain or very frightened of something and are using an immature way of dealing with their feelings. Either way, the nurse can be the target. When you are in someone else's home you are obviously on their territory, not yours, and that can leave you feeling very vulnerable. Most patients are grateful for the services which they are given by nurses, but the occasional patient can become either abusive or physically aggressive. It is not possible here to give any lengthy instructions for ways of dealing with violent or abusive patients, but one or two points are worth noting.

The first concern is that of safety: your own, and that of the patient. Most health authorities issue guidelines about the correct procedures to follow if there is any question of physical violence, and every nurse is advised to be familiar with these guidelines. They are aimed at ensuring that the threat of violence can be dealt with without it ever developing into something more serious.

A very human response to being threatened is to defend yourself, of which a corollary is 'attack is the best form of defence'. So the most natural thing to do, when someone starts to attack you, is to defend yourself. Yet this is often experienced by your attacker as an attack on him or her. Even if you did not mean it that way, you may make things worse. For instance, if you defend yourself by proclaiming your innocence, or pointing out that the patient may also be at fault in some way, the patient is likely to feel that you are being hostile and aggressive, too. So in return, the patient may well fight back. What happens is that the conflict escalates, which does no good to anyone.

The best way of handling the threat of attack in many instances may well be to do the thing which does *not* come naturally, and *avoid* jumping immediately to your defence. (Obviously we are not talking about instances where a physical assault has been made on you.) You can try to calm down the situation by *not* reacting to the threat. For example, you can tell the threatening person that you understand the way he or she feels, so would they please explain a bit more, so that you can try to help. This can have a remarkable effect on the threatening person. Instead of being faced by a hostile, unhelpful nurse they are faced by someone who is perhaps trying to be of assistance. This manoeuvre is not suitable for use with all people at all times, but it is worth a try, as it immediately calms the situation down. An alternative way of defusing possibly explosive situations is to acknowledge instantly the angry person's right to be angry, by telling the person that you feel that he or she is entitled to feel that way. Of course, you may not *actually* feel this way, but if your aim is to calm the situation down then this is a good first move.

You can only start to communicate effectively with people if both you and they are talking, not shouting. Therefore, your main aim must be to calm the person down and stay calm yourself. If you think that there is no hope of being able to do this then you should try to leave the situation as soon as you can, and if possible return later with a colleague who can act as a go-between. This is especially important if it is something that *you* have said or done which has apparently caused the anger.

Dealing with the seductive patient

The problem of the seductive patient may appear to be the opposite of the aggressive patient, but actually the two are not so different. Like the violent patient, the seductive patient is forcing his or her attentions on to you without your invitation or consent. The seriousness of the problem can vary. Sometimes it is simply the case of a patient or relative being a bit over-friendly, and turning a harmless flirtation into a not-so-harmless proposition. Such situations are best dealt with promptly and humorously, although this does not always mean they are easy situations to cope with. Some nurses may in fact wonder guiltily whether they in some way provoked the attention, and this can lead to an awful lot of heart-searching, often without cause. (This is where the support and back-up of the team is vital.) But sometimes patients, or relatives of patients, can be rather insistent, or even unpleasant in their approach. While many nurses may learn how to cope with this sort of proposition, it can be quite alarming when it first happens, and can seriously threaten the nurse's confidence.

There are a variety of ways of dealing with unwanted propositions, and most of us will have learnt these skills as part of normal growing up. But it is one thing to be approached by someone at a party, quite another being propositioned by a patient or relative in the person's own bedroom, when there is no one else in the house. One of the problems faced by young or inexperienced nurses is that they may feel very uneasy about asserting themselves, and saying 'no' loudly and clearly, thinking this to be rather impolite, or that they may hurt the other person's feelings. But being assertive is not the same thing as being aggressive. Being assertive is knowing your own rights, and having the confidence to stand up for them. The assertive person is able to say 'no' and mean it. Because of their fears of being thought aggressive, many people are frightened of being assertive, and so will say 'no' rather quietly and apologetically. Unfortunately, this is sometimes misinterpreted as meaning 'yes'. Although there will still be times when even the most assertive person in the world may still be a victim of sexual intimidation or attack, if you are self-confident and clear about what you want and what you do not want you can considerably reduce your chances of someone taking advantage of you.

An additional problem is of course the possibility of being accused by a patient of some indiscretion which you have not in fact committed. For example, a patient might complain that a nurse became over-familiar when carrying out some rather intimate procedure, such as a vaginal examination or catheter check. Alternatively, a patient might misinterpret a hug which was intended to be an encouragement as an attempted seduction. There are no easy answers to problems like these, as few nurses will want to restrict their professional practices because of a very small risk of being misunderstood. But there is one precaution that you can take which is relatively straightforward, and that is to explain to patients in detail what you are doing, and why. If you do this, they have at least some understanding of what your aims are and what your actions are for, so that there is less room for misunderstanding.

Being careful

It must be stressed that serious violent or sexual attacks by patients and relatives are not common. But these problems can be very frightening when you are on your own, miles away from the office or hospital. Knowing about the possibilities will not *prevent* such things from happening, but a few safeguards can cut down the possibility of them happening. If you do fear that either physical violence or sexual intimidation is on the cards, insist that two of you make visits together. If a patient or a relative appears to be becoming particularly attached to you, and you suspect that the interest is inappropriately intimate, then you should always insist on handing the case on to someone else (obviously explaining this to the patient in such a way as to avoid hurting too much). If you are really alarmed about the possibility of physical attack, you should get the full support of your team and ask a colleague to be present with you.

Whilst we do not want to overemphasize the dangers of working on your own, because it is the independence and responsibility which usually attracts nurses to community work, there are inevitably hazards of working alone which have been faced by most nurses working in the community. They all contribute to the experience of burnout which we described in Chapter 11, and they deserve to be taken seriously by nurses and nurse managers alike.

Taking responsibility

The second peril is this very independence and responsibility. Working in the community, away from either the hospital or department base, means that nurses have to face tricky situations which require instant decisions, with real consequences for patients but without adequate back-up. On occasion, nurses may even have to face situations of life and death. This can be extremely alarming, especially if the nurse is not prepared for them.

Louise, a district nurse, was one afternoon making a routine visit to an elderly gentleman who suffered from diabetes. When she arrived, she discovered that she could not open the front door. To her horror, she saw through the frosted glass of the door panel that something was lying on the floor of the hall, blocking the way. This 'something' looked very like the body of her patient. She had no key to open the door, so she quickly grabbed a piece of wood from the garden, and smashed the door panel.

*Inside, Louise saw her patient lying apparently unconscious on the floor.
She immediately checked his blood sugar levels, injected glucagon and
telephoned the practice to call for additional help, since she knew that
there were a number of further complications in the patient's history.
    When an ambulance arrived, the condition of her patient appeared to
have worsened, and he was dead on arrival at hospital. It turned out
that he had suffered from a coronary arythmia, probably worsened by his
diabetic condition. Louise thought long and hard about whether she had
acted in the right way, and whether there was anything else she should
or could have done. Understandably, the incident shook her. While all of
her colleagues tried to reassure her that she had done all she could have
done under the circumstances, she nevertheless felt both guilty and
shocked at the isolated nature of the old man's death, when she had been
a major source of human contact for him over many months.*

Other, less dramatic but equally disturbing incidents can happen when
patients ask for help that a nurse feels either unable or unwilling to give;
for instance, when a patient who has been discharged from hospital
suffering from a terminal illness such as cancer asks the nurse about the
diagnosis or prognosis of their disease. While many doctors now have a
policy of telling patients when they are dying, there are still some cases
where the patient may not know. Alternatively, the patient may have
been told, but is unwilling to accept the truth. In both these cases, the
nurse has to be extremely skillful in communicating with the patient,
especially if the nurse does not know what the patient knows.

The first thing to do is to find out exactly what the patient does or does
not know through careful and sensitive questioning. It is crucial to
remember that patients do not always understand medical jargon, so that
misunderstandings can often creep in. Sometimes these could be almost
comical, if they were not so painful for the patients concerned. Terms
which are familiar to the nurse may be unfamiliar to the patient; for
example, when we say 'chronic' we mean 'long-lasting', while for a
patient it may mean 'very serious'. And the word 'terminal' in some
contexts may mean 'the end of something' to us, while to a patient it may
mean 'leading to death'.

Having found out what the patient knows, the nurse has to decide
what to do next. We have already discussed the difficulties involved in
communication with the dying patient in Chapter 5. Patients will often
give clues about whether they are willing to discuss their condition and
are able to deal with bad news. Follow these clues. When you really do
not know what to say, remember that the nurse is in a very good position

to help the patient to explore feelings about the illness and the prognosis without necessarily having to 'tell all'. Consult colleagues and get some advice, though there will be times when you cannot afford to wait. At this point the nurse simply has to use his or her own professional skills, and make the best judgement possible under the circumstances. Being a professional means that you sometimes have to take risks and count on the soundness of your own judgement.

Some of the instances when you wish you were not out on your own occur when you reach the limits of your training (as in the examples that we described in Chapter 11). In some cases you may be able to help by finding some more information. Your inability to answer may come from a lack of knowledge, which is much easier to deal with than a lack of confidence in your skills. For example, when a patient asks you a question that you are unable to answer simply because you do not know the answer, then the best thing to do is to say so, and find out the answer later. In other cases, recognize the limitations of your own competence, and hand the case on to someone else. This can only be in the long-term interests of your patient. A patient might ask you to intervene in some family problem, or may ask you to treat some condition which has not been so far discussed with their doctor. In these cases, the appropriate course of action is to explain that you are not the best person to ask, but that Dr X at the surgery or Miss Y at social services can probably help. Patients are usually quite ready to recognize that no one nurse can know everything, and will accept that they may need to be referred on to someone else. But this should be explained to the patient, in language that they can understand. Remember that the one thing that patients say over and over again about their experience of nursing care is that they value being told what is happening to them, and why. If you are going to refer your patient on to someone else, then tell the patient when, why, and what to expect.

TAKING NURSING INTO THE COMMUNITY

In the last section of this chapter, we want to look briefly at the tremendous advantages of working in the community. Community nursing is very well placed to have an enormous impact on the welfare of countless thousands of patients each year. Because the nurse is working alone, in patients' homes, nursing care can be extended to all sorts of problems which otherwise might go unnoticed. But because the nurse also has a team in the background, a lot of support and skill exists which can be drawn upon if it is needed.

So what is special about the nurse in the community? There are at least four aspects of the job of community nursing which make it stand out as a particularly important part of health care, and which may help to explain the positive impact of nursing in the community.

The nurse's power to influence

For a start, nurses tend to be respected and welcomed figures, whose opinions are valued by their patients and their patients' relatives. The nurse therefore has a very considerable potential for influencing the overall standard of health in the general population. For example, the nurse's opinions on whether or not a patient should continue smoking during pregnancy are likely to be heeded more than a neighbour's, as most people assume that a nurse is an expert on these matters. It may be hard to accept that you are a figure of some influence and importance in your patients' lives, but the fact is that you are, and you therefore have enormous scope for increasing people's awareness of the need to lead healthier lives. Your qualifications, training and the uniform you wear all combine to give you status, which expertise underpins. But, in addition, we know that really effective nurses (like really effective teachers, social workers or doctors) add to this professionalism their own unique personal characteristics, such as a sense of humour, kindness or humane consideration for others. This means that the power and influence of the nurse is based on a combination of personal and professional qualities, both of which can be very well displayed in the setting of people's own homes.

The nurse in personal contact

Secondly, the fact that the nurse is in the community rather than in some rather remote office is enormously important. Despite the sums of money that are given to health education campaigns in the media, the really effective health education is that which takes place in the home. Personal contact is most important. For example, advice from a district nurse about the importance of regular physical exercise will have more impact when the district nurse in question is the person who calls every Tuesday afternoon, rather than the posh stranger on the television. No matter how 'insignificant' you may feel, if your patients like and respect you, you will actually have a more convincing effect on them than some famous media personality ever will.

The nurse and community care

Thirdly, it is now general health policy to shift the care of many groups of patients from large institutions into the community, and this includes psychiatric, mentally handicapped and elderly patients. This has already radically affected the workloads of many community nurses, and will undoubtedly mean that more time is spent with these types of patients in the future. But it also means that the key figure in the health care of many of our sick patients is going to be the community nurse. This pattern of care means that the personal responsibility carried by each individual community nurse is likely to increase considerably. So will the power of the community nursing services as a whole.

The nurse and prevention

Lastly, as the profession of nursing develops it seems likely that more emphasis will be placed on prevention rather than cure. The nurse in the community is in the best position to implement preventive health care strategies. Because community nurses go into people's homes, they are able to notice the things which might otherwise go unnoticed and unreported. In this way, the nurse can prevent numerous accidents or infections in the home, as well as teaching positive health values. Obviously it is easier to treat both physical and emotional distress if it is picked up early enough. The nurse in the community clearly has a key role here.

IN CONCLUSION

Throughout this book we have pointed out the ways in which the individual differences between people need to be recognized and respected by nurses working in the community. We have also shown that nurses have an enormous potential for improving the health and wellbeing of the patients who are referred to them by taking account of these individual needs and experiences. But we hope that we have also shown that the same applies to nurses themselves, who also deserve to be treated as unique individuals, with emotional and personal reactions of their own. If nursing services in the community choose to pay attention to the individual in this way, as well as to the physical needs of patients, then the profession is sure to grow and thrive to the benefit of patients and nurses alike. Neither nurses nor patients deserve any less.

Suggestions for further reading

Dickson, A. (1982) *A Woman in Your Own Right*. London: Quartet.
  Although written primarily for women, this book could benefit nurses of both sexes who wish they were more able to assert themselves comfortably in a

whole variety of situations. It includes a clear account of what being assertive entails, and tells you how to try to change your behaviour from being either aggressive or a door-mat for someone else to being assertive. It is well written and directly applicable to daily life.

Skevington, S. (1984) *Understanding Nurses: The social psychology of nursing.* Chichester: Wiley.
Each chapter is written by experts in different aspects of nursing; on conflict between different groups of nurses; the behaviour of ward sisters; and the role of male nurses. Also includes chapters on the personal experience of being either a patient or a nurse.

Zander, A. (1979) *Groups at Work.* San Francisco: Jossey Bass.
About groups at work, why they have problems, and how to get the best out of them.

Index

ABORTION, and nurses 87–90
abuse *see* child abuse
adopted children, and parenting 108–9
ageing
    attitudes to 19
    and blindness 34
    economic aspects 13–14
    and mental ability 8, 14
    positive aspects 18–19
    process 6–14
    reactions to 11–13
    and sex 8, 95
    social aspects 8–10
  see also elderly
aggression, dealing with 170–1
anger, patients' 50, 170–1
anxiety, and death 55–6
  see also stress
assessment of elderly 14–15
attitudes to death 54–5, 57–61
attitudes to mental handicap 24, 27–8

BEREAVEMENT
  coping with 65–6
  definition 63
  and elderly 12
  stages 63–5
blindness
  and ageing 34
  and mobility 34–5
bonding
  and adoption 108
  maternal 102
bowel control 43
breast, and women's identity 45–6
burnout
  avoidance 156–9

causes 149–55
definition 145–6
recognition 146–8

CARE, community *see* community care
carers
  and burnout 149
  and guilt 18
  and nurses 14–15, 17
  and stress 135–6
change
  bodily 99
  and family 69 *et seq.*
  and stress 133–4
child abuse
  definition 113–4
  emotional 121–3
  and nurses 113
  physical 114–7
  sexual 117–21
  see also child neglect
child neglect 123–6
children
  adopted 108–9
  and death 61–2
  and divorce 76
  emotional development 124
  handicapped, and parenting 109–11
  individual differences 1–5
  and limit-testing 109
colostomy *see* ostomy
communal family 70–1
communication
  and babies 104–5
  and blindness 35–6
  and conflict 165–6
  and deafness 33–4

and elderly 15–16
and family 72–3
and nurses 152, 158–9
and patients 174–5
community care
    and elderly 6, 13–14
    and mental handicap 23, 24
    nurses' role 176–7
    and terminal illness 53–4
conflict
    and communication 165–6
    group 164–7
context, importance of 4
contraception, and nurses 89
counselling, and bereavement 65
counselling skills, and nurses 16, 141–2
counsellors, nurse 157

DEAFNESS
    and communication 33–4
    social aspects 33–4
death
    and anxiety 55–6
    attitudes to 54–5, 57–61
    and children 61–2
    and depression 59
    and loneliness 56–7, 59
    and nurses 53–4
    nurses' attitudes 66–7
    and religious beliefs 67
depression
    and death 59
    and stress 130
dialysis, adjustment to 40–1
disabled, and sex 93–4
divorce
    and children 76
    and family 75
    reactions to 76–7
drugs, and stress 142–3

ECONOMIC ASPECTS of ageing 13–14
economic aspects of physical handicap
    31–2
education
    health, and nurses 175–7
    and parenting 98
elderly
    assessment of 14–15
    and bereavement 12
    and communication 15–16
    and community care 6, 13–14
    individual differences in 6–7
    and infantilization 16
    nursing skills with 14–18

and self-esteem 9, 11–12
emotional demands on nurses 149–50

FAILURE to thrive 124–5
family
    and change 69 *et seq.*
    communal 70–1
    and communication 72–3
    demands of 153–5
    and divorce 75
    involvement in treatment 51
    single parent 70–1
    and social mobility 73–4
    and step-parenting 77–9
family planning, and nurses 89
fathers, and parenting 103

GROUP CONFLICT 164–7
groups, and identity 162–4
guilt, and carers 18

HANDICAP, definition 21
handicapped, and sex 93–4
handicapped children, and parenting
    109–11
health education, and nurses 175–7
health services, conflict in 165
home, and stress 133–4
hospitalization, and stress 137–9

IDENTITY, and groups 162–4
ileostomy *see* ostomy
illness, and personality 3
individual differences 3
    and children 1–5
    and elderly 6–7
infantilization, and elderly 16
information, and patients 18, 136–7

KÜBLER-ROSS, E. 57

LEADERSHIP 169
lifestyle change, and treatment
    procedures 41 *et seq.*
limit-testing, and children 109
listening 16, 141–2, 169
loneliness, and death 56–7, 59
loss, and self-image 48

MASTECTOMY
    nurses' attitudes 46–8
    psychological aspects 44–5
    and self-image 45–6
masturbation 86, 94

maternal bonding 102
maternal instinct 100–1
mental ability, and ageing 8, 14
mental handicap
   attitudes to 24, 27–8
   causes 23–4
   and community care 23, 24
   definition 22
   and independence 29
   and nurses 25–8
   and prevention 25
   and sex 29
   and social skills 22–3, 28
   treatment 24–5
mental illness, definition 22
mobility, and blindness 34–5
mothers, working 103

NATURAL parenting 100–1
neglect, child 123–6
nurse counsellors 157
nurses
   and abortion 87–90
   attitudes to death 66–7
   attitudes to mastectomy 46–8
   and bereavement 65–6
   and burnout 145 *et seq.*
   and carers 14–15, 17
   and child abuse 113
   and communication 152, 158–9
   and contraception 89
   and counselling skills 16
   and death 53–4
   emotional demands 149–50
   and health education 175–7
   lack of training 151
   limits to helpfulness 50–2
   and mental handicap 25–8
   and patients' anger 50
   personal qualities 39
   and physical handicap 31–2
   and pregnancy counselling 87–90
   problems of working alone 170–5
   and professionalism 150
   and recognition 151–2
   and responsibility 173–5
   and sex education 87
   and sex roles 153
   and status 151–2, 176
   and stress 128 *et seq.*
   and work roles 153
nursing, as management 3
nursing skills, with elderly 14–18

OLD AGE *see* elderly

ostomy, social aspects 43–4

PAIN, fear of 55
parenting
   and adopted children 108–9
   causes of problems 99–100
   and fathers 103
   and handicapped children 109–11
   learning about 98
   natural 100–1
   and step-children 105–7
parents, needs of 111
patient care
   and conflict 166–7
   involvement of family 50
patients
   and communication 174–5
   and information 18, 136–7
   seductive 171–172
   special needs of 38
   violent 170–1
   as whole people 3
personal qualities of nurses 39
personality, and illness 3
physical exercise, and stress 141
physical handicap
   attitudes to 30–1
   causes 30
   economic aspects 31–2
   and nurses 31–2
   social aspects 31–2
   and stigma 30–1
physiological reaction to stress 129–30
play as conversation 105
pregnancy counselling, and nurses
   87–90
problem-sharing 141–2
problem-solving 42–3
professionalism, and nurses 150
propositions, unwanted 171–2
psychological reaction to stress 130–1

RELAXATION training 139–40
religious beliefs, and death 67
respect 16
responsibility, and nurses 173–5
retirement, reactions to 10–11
role, and self-image 39–40

SEDUCTIVE patients 171–2
self-esteem, and elderly 9, 11–12
self-help groups 141–2
self-image 39–40
   and loss 48
   and mastectomy 45–6

Selye, Hans 129
sensory handicap *see* blindness, deafness
separation, and family 73–4
sex
   and ageing 8, 95
   attitudes to 86–7
   and disabled 93–4
   and handicapped 93–4
   ignorance about 85–6
   and mental handicap 29
   and responsibility 87
   talking about 83–4
sex education, and nurses 87
sex roles
   and family 70, 101
   and nurses 153
sexual abuse, child 117–21
sexual difficulties 91–3
sexually transmitted diseases 96
single parent family 70–1
social aspects of ageing 8–10
social aspects of physical handicap 31–2
social mobility, and family 73–4
social skills, and mental handicap
      22–3, 28
special needs 39 *et seq.*
staff problems, and burnout 148, 150–1
stepchildren, and parenting 105–7
step-parenting, and family 77–9
stereotypes, and group conflict 165
stereotyping 49–50
stigma, and physical handicap 30–1
stress
   and carers 135–6
   causes 131–8
   definition 129
   and depression 130
   and drugs 142–3
   and hospitalization 137–9

   and nurses 128 *et seq.*
   and personal change 133–4
   physiological reaction 129–30
   psychological reaction 130–1
   stages 130
   and understanding 136–7
   and unemployment 134
   and work 131–2
   see also burnout
stress management 139–43, 156–9
suicide, effects of 81

TEAM WORK *see* groups
terminal illness
   and communication 174–5
   and community care 53–4
   emotional demands 152
thrive, failure to 124–5
training, nurses' lack of 151
tranquillizers, and stress 142–3
treatment
   importance of context 4
   involvement of family 51
treatment procedures, and lifestyle
      change 41 *et seq.*

UNDERSTANDING
   and anxiety 3–4
   and stress 136–7
unemployment, and stress 134

VENEREAL disease 96
violent patients 170–1

WHOLE PERSON, patient as 3
women's identity, and breast 45–6
work, and stress 131–2
work roles, and nurses 153
working mothers 103